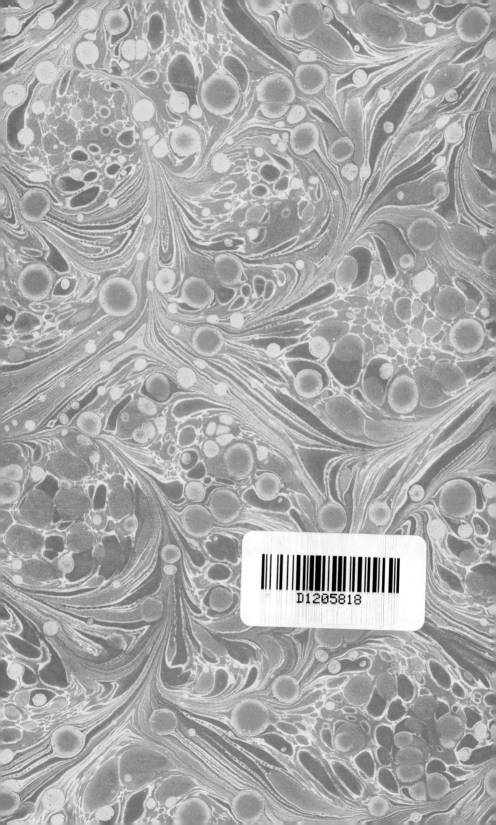

D1205818

This special edition of

ON

MALFORMATIONS, &c.,

OF THE

HUMAN HEART

By THOMAS B. PEACOCK, M.D.

has been privately printed

for the members of

The Classics of Medicine Library

ON

MALFORMATIONS, &c.,

OF THE

HUMAN HEART.

WITH ORIGINAL CASES.

LONDON :
RICHARD BARRETT, PRINTER,
MARK LANE.

ON

MALFORMATIONS, &c.,

OF THE

HUMAN HEART.

WITH ORIGINAL CASES.

BY

THOMAS B. PEACOCK, M.D.,

FELLOW OF THE ROYAL COLLEGE OF PHYSICIANS,

ASSISTANT-PHYSICIAN TO ST. THOMAS'S HOSPITAL, AND

PHYSICIAN TO THE HOSPITAL FOR DISEASES OF THE CHEST, VICTORIA PARK

LONDON:

JOHN CHURCHILL, NEW BURLINGTON STREET.

1858.

PREFACE.

SEVERAL examples of malformation of the heart having fallen under my notice, I have been induced for several years to pay special attention to this branch of medical science; and in 1854, shortly after an interesting case of malformation had occurred at St. Thomas's Hospital, I delivered a series of lectures on the subject to the students of that medical school. These lectures were subsequently published in the "Medical Times and Gazette;" and, together with several cases which have been at various times contributed to different medical societies and journals, are now reprinted, after the whole has been carefully revised and considerably extended.

There are few subjects which have attracted more attention in the profession than the irregularities in the development of the heart and large vessels. Longer or shorter notices of the chief varieties of malformation are contained in the different works on Morbid Anatomy, and in the systematic treatises on cardiac affections by Burns, Corvisart, Bertin, Laennec, Bouilland, and Hope. They have been made the subject of a special essay by Dr. Farre,[1] and of shorter memoirs by Dr. Paget,[2] Dr. Williams,[3]

[1] On Malformations of the Human Heart. London. 1814.
[2] On the Congenital Malformations of the Human Heart. Edin. Med. and Surg. Journ. vol. 36, 1831, p. 263.
[3] Cyclopædia of Practical Medicine, vol. 3, 1834, p. 65.

Dr. Todd,[1] Dr. Joy,[2] and Dr. Craigie ; by Haase,[4] Meckel,[5] and Hein ;[6] and by Louis[7] and Gintrac.[8] More recently the subject has been discussed in graduation theses by MM. Deguise[9] and Pize,[10] and in a series of valuable and interesting papers by Dr. Chevers.[11]

It might thus appear that there was scarcely scope for a new work in this department of pathology.   Several of the memoirs, however, which I have named were published at a period when the defects in the conformation of the heart were less studied than, in conjunction with other branches of morbid anatomy, they have recently been.   Others are limited to one department of the subject, and the treatise of Dr. Farre is professedly

[1] Cyclopædia of Anatomy and Physiology, vol. 2, 1839, p. 630.

[2] Library of Medicine, vol. 3, 1840, p. 381.

[3] Edin. Med. and Surg. Journ., vol. 60, 1843, Case of Cyanosis, or Blue Disease, etc.

[4] Dissertatio Inauguralis Medica de Morbo Cœruleo. Lipsiæ, 1813.

[5] De cordis conditionibus abnormibus Dissertatio Inauguralis. Halæ, 1802. Beitrag zur Geschichte der Bildungsfehler des Herzens welche die Bildung des rothen Blutes hindern. Deutsches Archiv f. d. Physiologie, Halle und Berlin, 1815, p. 221.

[6] De istis cordis deformationibus quæ sanginem venosum cum arterioso misceri permittunt. Gœttingæ, 1816.

[7] Observations et Recherches sur la Cyanose, ou Maladie Bleue. Paris, 1824.

[8] Archives Générales de Médecine, 2me serie, t. 3, 1823 ; Mémoires ou Recherches Anatomico-Pathologiques. Paris, 1826, p. 300.

[9] De la Cyanose Cardiaque, etc. Thèse de Paris, 1843.

[10] Considérations sur les Anomalies Cardiaques et Vasculaires qui peuvent Causer la Cyanose. These de Paris, 1854.

[11] Collection of Facts illustrative of Morbid Conditions of the Pulmonary Artery, London, 1851, originally published in London Medical Gazette, 1845 to 1851.   The causation of cyanosis is also discussed by Ferrus in the art. Cyanose, Dict. de Méd. 2me ed., t. 9, 1835, p. 527 ; by Stillé on Cyanosis or Morbus Cæruleus, in Am. Jour. of Med. Sc., N.S., vol. 8, Phil. 1844, p. 25 ; and by Copland, in the Dictionary of Practical Medicine, art. Blue Disease, vol. 1, p. 199.

incomplete. I have, therefore, thought that a work containing the more recent information, and regarding the subject in a practical point of view, would not be without interest and value to the profession.

The subjects treated of in the following essay embrace :—

I. Congenital Misplacements of the Heart.

II. Deficiency of the Pericardium.

III. Malformations of the Heart, including,

1st. Malformations dependent on arrest of development at an early period of fœtal life.

2ndly. Malformations preventing the changes which should ensue after birth; and,

3rdly. Malformations which do not interfere with the functions of the heart, but may lay the foundations of disease in after life.

IV. Malformations consisting in the irregular development of the primary vessels.

V. Mode of formation ; Symptoms and Effects ; Diagnosis and Medical Management of cases of malformation.

In the Essay it has been my aim to present the subject in a practical point of view, and I have therefore made no allusion to those forms of defect in the development of the heart which are incompatible with the existence of extra-uterine life, or which have only been met with in the lower animals. I have also endeavoured to apportion the space devoted to the description of the various malformations, to the relative frequency and importance of the several forms, and it will be found that some of them have been treated differently and at greater length than by former writers. The medical periodicals, especially of France and England, abound in cases of malformation. I have, however, not thought it desirable to quote many of these at length, but have preferred to allude concisely to those which formed the earliest published examples of each form of defect, or which presented some rare and remarkable deviation, and have generally contented myself with referring to the periodicals and other publications in which the more recent or ordinary cases are reported. A brief inspection of the numerous references cited, will show that to have quoted more extensively would have greatly swelled the bulk of the volume.

Those who desire to investigate the subject further, I may refer to the original sources of information here indicated; or to the essay of M. Gintrac, the theses of M. Deguise and M. Pize, and the papers of Dr. Chevers; in one or other of which, but particularly the latter, a large proportion of the cases, only briefly noticed or alluded to in this work, will be found quoted at length.

TABLE OF CONTENTS.

Plate 1, Seat and Form of Apertures in the Septum of the Ventricles.

Fig. 1, drawing of the left ventricle of the heart in the case exhibited at the Pathological Society by Dr. Quain ; removed from a youth 18 years of age ; referred to at pp. 25.

Figs. 2 and 3, drawings of portions of the heart in the case of Dr. Oldham— described at p. 25 and 45.

Fig. 2 exhibits the aperture in the septum of the ventricles as viewed from the right ventricle, and shows the communication with the *sinus* of the right ventricle.

Fig. 3 displays the form of the valvular apparatus of the pulmonary artery. The curtains are only two in number, but the larger valve displays the remains of division, in the form of a frenum or band extending from the edge of the valve to the side of the vessel.

The preparation of this heart is numbered B 11 in the Museum of the Hospital for Diseases of the Chest, Victoria Park. It was removed from a child 17 months old.

PLATE 1.

Fig.1.

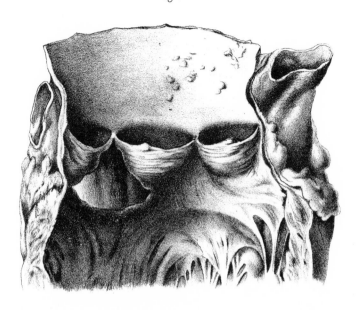

Fig.2.

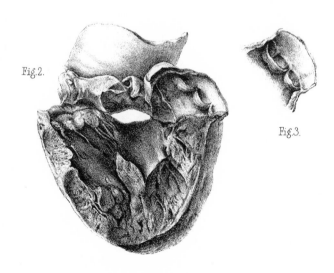

Fig.3.

Plate 2.—Obstruction at the Orifice of the Pulmonary Artery, and defect in the Septum Ventriculorum.

Fig. 1. Drawing of the heart described at p. 36.

The preparation is marked B 4, in the Museum of the Victoria Park Hospital. The child was 2 years and 5 months old.

a. The right ventricle laid open.

b. The contracted aperture of the pulmonary artery.

c. The left ventricle.

d. The ascending aorta.

The bristles passed into the aorta from behind and visible above the upper edge of the vessel, are seen to pass into both ventricles.

Fig. 2. Form of the valves of the pulmonary artery in this specimen.

Figs. 3 and 4 display the form of the valvular apparatus in the case of Mr. Marshall, described at p. 41.

The preparation is numbered B 6 in the Museum of the Victoria Park Hospital. The boy who was the subject of this malformation was 6½ years of age.

Fig. 3 exhibits the valves as seen from above, or from the pulmonary artery.

Fig. 4, with the coats supposed to be divided so as to show, the peculiar infundibular or barrel-shaped aperture from the ventricle into the artery.

PLATE. II.

Fig.1.

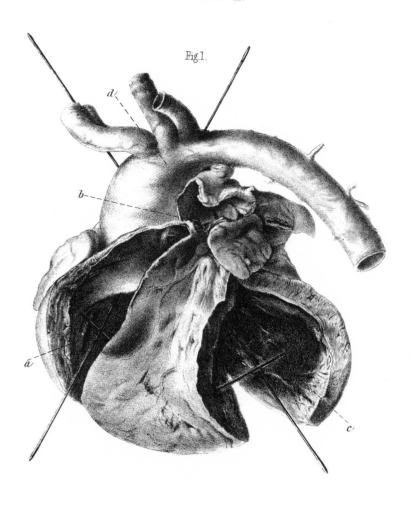

Fig.4.

Fig.2.   Fig 3

Tuffen West del. et lith. ad nat.   W. West Imp.

Plate 3.—Obstruction at the Orifice of the Pulmonary Artery and open Foramen Ovale.

Figs. 1 and 2. Drawings of portions of the heart in the case described at p. 83. The preparation is numbered B 3 in the Museum of the Victoria Park Hospital. The septum of the ventricles is entire, yet the hypertrophy of the right ventricle is seen to be very great. The young woman who was the subject of the disease died at the age of 20.

    a. The right ventricle laid open to show the great hypertrophy of its parietes.

    b. The pulmonic orifice.

Fig. 2. The orifice of the pulmonary artery as seen from above. The union of the three valves into one, the frena or bands which mark the former division of the segments, the thickening of the whole of the valves, and the form of the orifice, are well shown in this drawing.

Fig. 3. The foramen ovale in the same case, showing that the process of closure has never been completed, the cornua of the valve, *a, a,* still remaining widely apart.

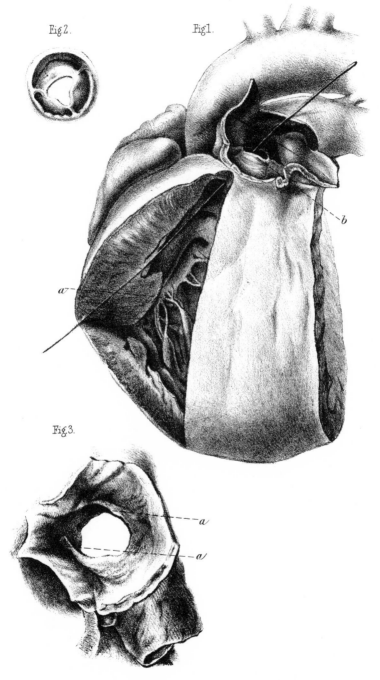

PLATE III

Fig 2.

Fig 1.

b

a

Fig. 3.

- - - *a*

- - - *a*

Tuffen West del. et lith. ad nat.

W. West Imp.

Plate 4.—Obstruction and Obliteration of the Orifice of the Pulmonary Artery.

Fig. 1. Form of the valvular apparatus in the specimen referred to at p. 35, existing in the Museum of St. Thomas's Hospital and numbered 1437. It has probably been removed from a young person 9 or 10 years of age.

Fig. 2. Drawing of obstruction at the orifice of the pulmonary artery, as existing in the case described at p. 42.

The preparation is marked B 7 in the Victoria Park Museum. It was removed from a girl 19 years of age.

The valves are seen to be two in number, and are of considerable size, the obstruction being situated in their bases or at the exit from the ventricle.

The open ductus arteriosus in this case is shown in plate 5, fig. 1.

Fig. 3. Obliteration of the trunk of the pulmonary artery ; pulmonary branches supplied through the ductus arteriosus. Case described at p. 56.

The child which was the subject of the malformation died when nearly one year old, and the specimen is numbered B 8 in the Museum of the Victoria Park Hospital.

a. Right ventricle.

b. Left ventricle.

c. Ascending aorta.

d. The obliterated trunk of pulmonary artery.

e. The open ductus arteriosus.

f, f. The pulmonary branches.

PLATE IV.

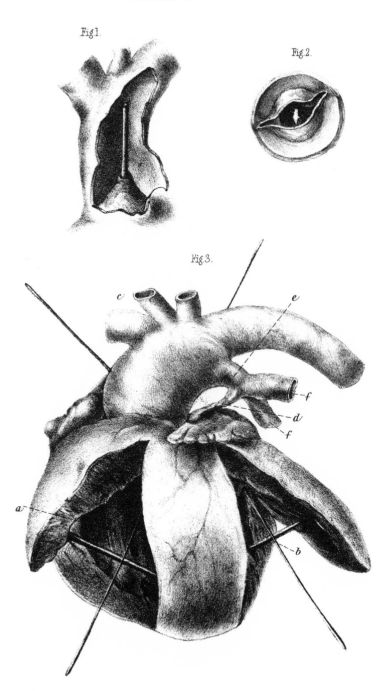

Fig 1.

Fig. 2.

Fig. 3.

c

e

f

d

f

a

b

Tuffen West del. et lith. ad nat.   W. West Imp.

Plate 5.—Open Ductus Arteriosus and Supernumerary Septum in the Right Ventricle.

Fig. 1. Showing the situation of the open ductus arteriosus, *a*, in the case described at p. 42.

The form of the pulmonic obstruction in this case is seen in plate 4, fig. 2.

In the two last specimens the ductus arteriosus is seen to be inserted into the aorta at a higher part than is usual at the time of birth.

Fig. 2. Supernumerary septum in the right ventricle, as existing in the case described at p. 68.

The child died of hemorrhage during scarlatina, when 5 years of age.

The specimen is marked B 2 in the Victoria Park Hospital Museum.

a. Sinus of right ventricle laid open.

b. Infundibular portion of right ventricle.

c. Opening in supernumerary septum.

PLATE V

Fig.1.

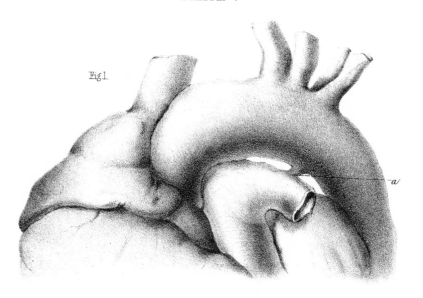

a

Fig.2.

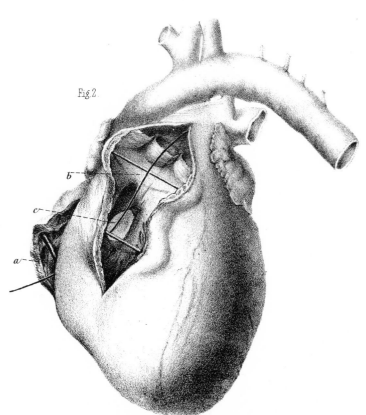

b

c

a

Tuffen West del.et lith.ad nat.   W.West Imp.

Plate 6.—Supernumerary Septum in the Right Ventricle and open Foramen Ovale.

Fig. 1. Supernumerary septum in right ventricle with deficiency of the interventricular septum and contraction of the pulmonic orifice. From a youth aged 15, whose case is described at p. 63. The preparation is numbered B 5 in the Museum of the Victoria Park Hospital.

  a. Sinus of the ventricle greatly hypertrophied.

  b. Infundibular portion.

  c. Valvular apparatus, and trunk of pulmonary artery obstructed by coagula.

  d. Opening in the supernumerary septum.

  e. Left ventricle.

Fig. 2. Aperture in the septum of the auricles in the situation of the foramen ovale, but without any valve. From a preparation in St. Thomas's Hospital Museum, numbered 579, said to have been removed from a girl 13 or 14 years of age. See pp. 78 and 85.

Fig. 3. Open foramen ovale in case referred to at pp. 78 and 86. The preparation was removed from a girl aged 8, and is numbered B 16 in the Museum of the Victoria Park Hospital.

PLATE VI.

Fig.1.

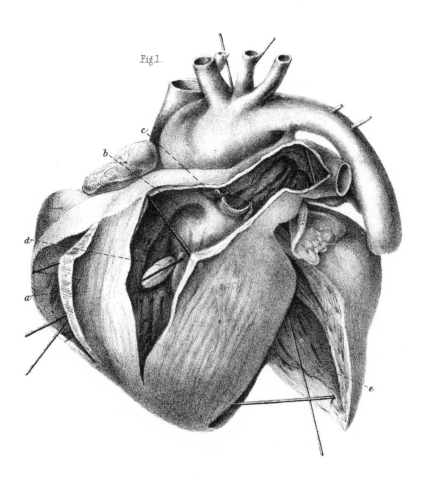

c

b

d

a

e

Fig 2

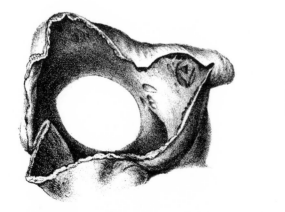

Fig.3.

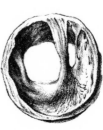

J.Perry & T.W. del   Tuffen West lith.   W.West.Imp.

Plate 7.—Defect in the Number of the Semilunar Valves.

Fig. 1. Fusion of two of the aortic valves, from a child 10 weeks old, whose case is described at p. 108, Dr. Rees' patient. There was a contraction of the aorta distal to the left subclavian artery and an open ductus arteriosus. The case was therefore one of descending aorta partly given off from the pulmonary artery. The preparation is marked B 17 in the Museum, Victoria Park Hospital.

Fig. 2. Similar specimen removed from a boy, aged 15, who was crushed to death.

It is numbered B 14 in the Museum of the Victoria Park Hospital.

In both these specimens the frenum or band, marking the former point of union, is well seen in the larger valve.

Fig. 3. Drawing from a preparation, marked β 110, in St. Thomas's Hospital Museum. The frenum or band on the upper side of the larger valve cannot be seen in this view ; but the sulcus is well marked below.

Fig. 4. Drawing exhibiting the form of defect, in which one valve, a, has become atrophied from disease in fœtal or early life ; the larger valves b, b, also exhibit the effects of subsequent disease so often seen in these cases. From a preparation marked β 69 in St. Thomas's Hospital Museum, removed from a man 60 years of age.

PLATE VII.

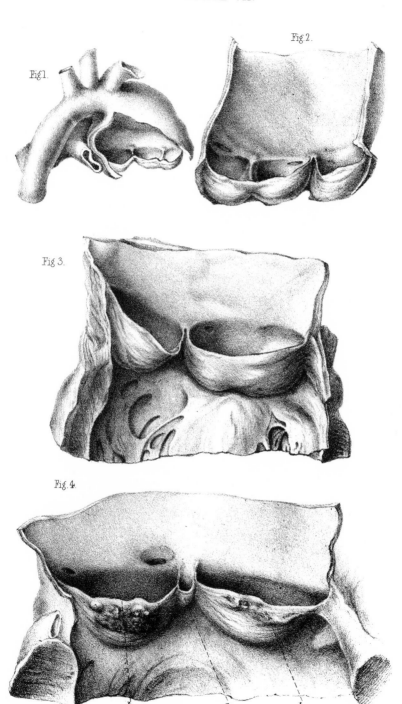

Fig 1.

Fig 2.

Fig 3.

Fig. 4.

b   *a*   *b*

Tuffen West del. et lith. ad nat.   W. West Imp.

Plate 8.—Excess in the number of the Semilunar Valves.

Fig. 1. Four valves at the orifice of the pulmonary artery, the excess being apparently produced by the division of one of the valves at *a*. The two segments so produced are imperfect and are freely blended together. From a female 75 years of age. The preparation is numbered B 13, in the Museum of the Victoria Park Hospital.

Fig. 2. Four valves at the orifice of the pulmonary artery; the excess consisting in three imperfectly divided segments and one complete segment. The larger fold at *a, a*, is attached to the side of the vessel by firm bands. From a man, 45 years of age, who was crushed to death.

Fig. 3. Four valves at the aortic orifice, from a preparation in St. Thomas's Hospital Museum, numbered β 105. The excess is apparently due to the division of one fold at *a* into two. The septum between these two segments is very imperfect, being, as seen in fig. 4, perforated by apertures, or displaying portions in which the fibrous tissue is wanting. It is doubtful whether the small body marked *b*, fig. 3, is an adhesion between the curtains or a supernumerary valve.

Fig. 5. Five valves at the orifice of the pulmonary artery, from a preparation marked B 12 in Museum of the Victoria Park Hospital, removed from a child aged 4½ years. The excess is apparently due to the division of two curtains at *a* and *b*. The supernumerary segments and those adjacent to them are imperfect.

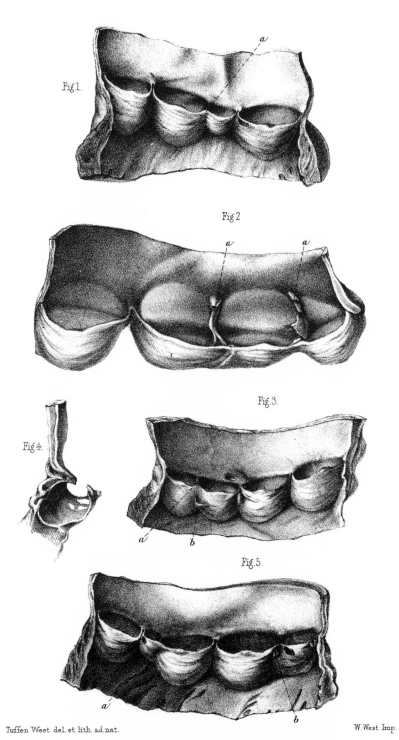

PLATE VIII.

Fig 1.

a

Fig 2

a   a

Fig 3.

Fig 4.

a'   b

Fig. 5.

a'

b

Tuffen West del. et lith. ad. nat.   W. West Imp.

I.

MISPLACEMENTS OF THE HEART.

THE heart may be congenitally misplaced in various ways, occupying either an unusual position within the thorax, or being situated external to that cavity.

Transposition.

The most frequent of the internal misplacements is that in which the heart is placed in a similar position on the right side of the chest to that which it should occupy on the left. When this occurs, the viscera of the body generally are also most usually transposed; but such is not always the case, the heart being occasionally situated on the right side, while the other viscera retain their usual positions. M. Breschet in his memoir,[1] states that he has seen four instances of this displacement of the heart in newly born children, in whom the other viscera occupied their natural positions.

When the heart is transposed to the right side, it may be well-formed, as in the cases related by Dr. Sampson,[2] M. Méry,[3] Dr. Baillie,[4] M. J. F. Meckel,[5] and M. Bosc.[6] The arteries also may be misplaced relatively to the ventricles, as in a case reported by Mr. Gamage.[7] Or the heart may be very imperfectly developed, and

[1] Sur l'Ectopie de l'appareil de la Circulation et particulièrement sur celle du Cœur ; Rep. Gén. D'Anat. et de Phys. Pathol., t. 2, 1826, p. 1.

[2] Phil. Trans. for the year 1674, vol. 9, No. 107, p. 146.

[3] Hist. de l'Acad. Royale des Sc., t. 2, 1686 to 1699 ; Paris, 1733, p. 44 ; observation contributed in 1688.

[4] Phil. Trans., 1788, pt. 1, p. 350 ; Works by Wardrop, vol. 1, p 148.

[5] De Cordis conditionibus abnormibus, Dissertatio inauguralis, Halæ, 1802, Tab. 1 and 4.

[6] Bullet. de la Soc. Anat. de Paris, an. 4, 1829, p. 42.

[7] New England Journal of Medicine and Surgery, vol. 4, 1815, p. 244.

the vessels arising from its cavities or entering into them, may be irregular, as in cases related by Breschet,[1] Martin,[2] and Boyer.[3]

Though a considerable number of instances of transposition of the heart have been observed, I have not myself had the opportuntity of examining any case of the kind after death. In 1849, however, a boy presented himself at the City Hospital for Diseases of the Chest, in whom the heart was placed on the right side, its apex beating an inch and a half below the right nipple, while the liver was situated on the left side. He had been an invalid since he was three years old, and, although then eighteen years of age, he looked like a much younger person, and had a peculiar sickly, unhealthy appearance.

The heart may also be placed in the *median line* of the chest, and of this form of misplacement M. Breschet gives an instance which will again be referred to as an example of defective development of the organ. That writer also admits the existence of displacements in the *transverse* and *antero-posterior directions*, but gives no examples of either of these forms.

Exposition.

The most remarkable deviations from the natural position of the heart are, however, those in which the organ is situated wholly or in part external to the thoracic cavity ; and of this form three varieties are admitted, to which the terms Ectopia Pectoralis, E. Ventralis, and E. Cephalica have been given.

Ectopia Pectoralis Cordis (*Weese*).—This form of misplacement may occur either without any defect or fissure of the thoracic parietes or with such imperfections. As examples, Breschet refers to cases by Shulz and Vaubonnais, in which the misplacement existed in fœtuses; to others, by Buttner and Weese, in a child which lived thirty-six to forty hours; by Martinez, in which life was prolonged twelve hours; and by Sandifort, in which the child survived for a day. Alone, this form of malformation is rare ; but when the viscera of the abdomen also are protruded, it is not of uncommon occurrence. Cases

---

[1] Op. Cit., 1re obs., p. 7.

[2] Breschet, Op. Cit., 2me obs., p. 9 ; and Bullet. de la Soc. Anat., 1826, p. 39.

[3] Arch. Gén. de Méd., 4me serie, t. 23, 1850, p. 90 ; and Gaz. Méd. de Paris, 20me an., t. 5, 1850, p. 292.

have more recently been related by Dr. O'Bryan,[1] Mr. Barrett,[2] Mr. Mitchell,[3] M. Follin,[4] and Mr. Sydney Jones.[5]

Ectopia Cordis Ventralis (Weese).—Of this form of misplacement there are also two varieties. In one, the heart is protruded through the diaphragm without forming a tumour externally; in the other, there is an external tumour. As examples of the first kind, M. Breschet refers to the case of Ramel, in which a female, ten years of age, had the heart situated immediately below the diaphragm. A much more remarkable instance is that related by M. Deschamps of Laval, of a man who had served in the army, and retired in consequence of suffering from severe pains in the loins. He, however, married, and had three children; but the lumbar pains continued, he became emaciated, and died exhausted by continued suffering. On examination, the right kidney was found large, hard, and in a state of suppuration; and a solid mass containing a cavity filled with sanies was situated in the pelvis. The heart occupied the place of the right kidney, and the vessels arising from it passed through an opening in the diaphragm into the thorax.

Of the second variety, the case of Mr. Wilson, to be hereafter mentioned, and others by Prochaska, Klein, Sandifort, &c., afford examples.

Ectopia Cordis Cephalica (Breschet).—In this form of displacement, the heart lies in the front of the neck, in connexion with the ramus of the jaw. In the only cases on record the malformation existed in foetuses, or in infants which scarcely survived birth and which presented other serious defects. It is therefore much less important than the other forms.

The two most interesting cases of misplacement which have been published since the appearance of M. Breschet's memoir are those of Dr. O'Bryan and Mr. Sydney Jones.

In the former case, the zyphoid cartilage was deficient, together with the fibres of the diaphragm inserted into that body;

---

[1] Prov. Med. and Surg. Trans., vol. 6, 1837, p. 374.

[2] Lancet, 1835. [3] Dublin Jour., vol. 26, 1844, p. 262.

[4] Arch. Gén. de Méd., 4me serie, t. 24, 1850, p. 101, and Gaz. Méd. de Paris, 1850. [5] Path. Trans., vol. 6, 1854–5, p. 98.

a triangular aperture was thus left, through which a portion of the left ventricle, covered with pericardium, was protruded, so as to form a soft, oval, unequal and semi-transparent tumour, at the anterior and upper part of the abdomen. The part of the left ventricle protruded was one inch and three-quarters in length, and a further portion was prevented escaping by the apex of the right ventricle. The lower part of the tumour was occupied by a portion of colon. The child survived three months, and died of bronchitis brought on by exposure.

In Mr. Sydney Jones' case the specimen was exhibited at the Pathological Society in 1855. The child was believed to have been born at the eighth month, and it survived thirteen hours. The heart, devoid of pericardium, was situated wholly external to the thoracic cavity. A fissure existed in the sternum of an oval shape, its longer diameter being nearly vertical and three-quarters of an inch in length, and its shorter diameter transverse and half an inch long. Through this opening the vessels passed from the heart into the thorax. The margin of the fissure was obscured anteriorly by a prolongation of skin on the great vessels, and from thence on the external surface of the heart. The cuticle could be traced as far as the base of the viscus and slightly over the auricles; but beyond this point there was no epithelial covering,—the muscular substance being only protected by a structure shown on microscopical examination to be a white fibrous, mixed with yellow, elastic tissue. The closing up of the foramen was completed posteriorly by the reflexion of the pleura from the great vessels on to the parietes of the thorax. The heart appears to have been well formed, and the child presented no other defect.

In the museum of St. Thomas' Hospital there is a specimen which affords an example of partial ectopia abdominalis. There is an aperture in the diaphragm three inches in diameter, at the edges of which the pericardium and peritoneum are perfectly continuous, and through this opening the apex and lower part of the heart protrudes, so that the organ is situated partly in the pericardial and partly in the peritoneal cavity. The heart rests upon the left lobe of the liver, which to some extent closes the defect in the diaphragm. A large portion of the great

omentum is situated within the pericardial sac, and is attached
by adhesions to the lower half of the anterior surface of the
heart, and to the corresponding part of the reflected pericardium. Considerable portions of the heart and of the orifice
are free from attachments, so that the finger might be readily
passed from the pericardium through the opening to the upper
surface of the left lobe of the liver. The preparation was
removed from the body of a man, a labourer, forty-seven years
of age, who died of gangrene and inflammation of the lung, with
chronic ulceration of the fauces.[1]

[1] For reference to various cases of misplacement of the heart, see Otto's
Pathological Anatomy (South's Translation), pp. 274–6.

II.

DEFICIENCY OF THE PERICARDIUM.

WHEN the heart is much misplaced, it is very generally deprived of its pericardial covering, as in some of the instances before referred to. Occasionally, also, the sac is wanting, when the organ occupies its natural position and is otherwise well formed.

Instances of the asserted absence of the pericardium have not unfrequently been recorded; yet it is probable that in some of these cases the membrane has not been really wanting, but only universally adherent, and that true congenital absence of the pericardium is of rare occurrence. One of the earliest authentic examples of this defect is that which occurred to Dr. Baillie,[1] in 1788; though that writer refers to cases related by Columbus, Bartholinus, and Littre, and to one mentioned in the Philosophical Transactions for 1740.[2] Dr. Baillie states that, on opening the cavity of the chest of a man 40 years of age, who had not presented any symptoms referable to the heart, in order to explain to his class the situation of the thoracic viscera, he was exceedingly surprised to find the heart lying naked in the left side. It was bare and distinct, and lay loose in the left cavity of the chest, unconnected in any way, except by its vessels; but was somewhat large, and was situated at a lower level than usual. The mediastinum consisted of two layers of pleura, united by cellular tissue. The right phrenic nerve ran between the laminæ of the mediastinum, near the right side of the heart, and the left phrenic nerve was

[1] Transactions of a Society for the Improvement of Medical and Surgical Knowledge, vol. 1, 1791, p. 91; and Works by Wardrop, vol. 1, p. 44.

[2] See also references in Otto's Pathological Anatomy (South's translation), p. 254, sects. 3 and 4.

situated between the same layers, almost immediately under the sternum.

In 1826, M. Breschet[1] described a similar defect, which was found in a man 28 years of age, who died of acute dysentery, under the care of M. Pettit. He had previously enjoyed good health. The heart was found lying loose in the left pleural sac, except that there existed adhesions between the base of the left ventricle and the left lung, and the apex of the heart and the diaphragm. The specimen was exhibited at the Académie de Médécine, and was examined by Cruveilhier, Laennec, Blainville, &c.

In 1839, a similar malformation fell under the notice of Mr. T. B. Curling,[2] in the body of a man aged 46, who died of paraplegia, at the London Hospital. He was not known to have manifested any peculiarity in the circulation. The heart occupied its natural position. There were some opaque spots on its surface, and the corresponding portions of the pleura covering the lungs were opaque and thickened.

In 1851, Dr Baly[3] exhibited at the Pathological Society, a specimen removed from a man 32 years of age, who died of phthisis, in the Millbank Penitentiary. He had never exhibited any symptoms of "obstructed or disordered circulation." The heart had no separate sac, and was in contact with the left lung, but not attached to the diaphragm. The left side of the heart and the left lung displayed some recent false membrane, and there was a slight adhesion between the apex of the heart and the lung. The left pleura was reflected over the heart and vessels, and then passed forwards to the sternum, and was there separated from the corresponding portion of the right pleura only by a thick layer of fibrous and cellular tissue. There was a rudimentary pericardium, in the form of a crescentic fold of the serous membrane, reflected beneath and behind the heart. This "fold, thickened by fibrous tissue between its layers, arose on the right side of the ascending aorta, passed

[1] Sur un Vice de Conformation Congéniale des Enveloppes du Cœur. Rep. d'Anat. et de Phys. Path., vol. 1, p. 67.

[2] Med.-Chir. Trans. N. S., vol. 2, p. 22.

[3] Path. Trans., vol. 3, 1850-51, 51-52, p. 60.

downwards to the right of the right auricle, and in front of the inferior vena cava, and, crossing behind the left auricle, terminated in the left pulmonary veins." A similar fold of membrane, representing the rudimentary pericardium, is noticed as having existed in the cases of M. Breschet and Mr. Curling. In both Mr. Curling's and Dr. Baly's cases, the left phrenic nerve passed to the right of the heart, between the layers of pleura forming the mediastinum.

In Dr. Baly's case, I had the opportunity of examining the specimen at the Pathological Society, and, some time previously, an instance of partial deficiency of the pericardium fell under my notice. The heart was separated from the right pleural sac by a layer of serous membrane covering a fibrous septum, while on the left side it lay loose in the cavity of the pleura, in connexion with the lung, with which it had contracted adhesions. From the circumstances under which the post-mortem examination was performed, I was not able to examine the parts so carefully as would have been desirable. The subject of the case was a man 75 years of age, who died of aortic valvular disease. In the other cases mentioned, the heart was healthy.

III.

MALFORMATIONS OF THE HEART.

1. MALFORMATIONS DEPENDANT ON ARREST OF DEVELOPMENT AT AN EARLY PERIOD OF FŒTAL LIFE.

HEART CONSISTING OF TWO CAVITIES.

HEARTS consisting of only two cavities, an auricle and a ventricle, with a single vessel supplying both the systemic and pulmonic circulations, have, though rarely, been found in infants which have survived for a short period after birth.[1] If we except the cases of Pozzi[2] and Lanzoni,[3] which are too imperfectly described to be relied upon, the first instance of this description of malformation was related to the Royal Society by Mr. Wilson in 1798.[4] Since that time an example of biloculate heart occurred to Dr. Farre in 1814,[5] and a specimen was presented to the Pathological Society by Mr. Foster in 1846.[6] A heart exhibiting a somewhat more advanced degree of development was described by Mr. Standert,[7] in the Philosophical Transactions for 1805, and a similar case was met with at Philadelphia, by Mr. Mauran, in 1827,[8] and others have since been described by M. Thore,[9] Dr. Crisp,[10] Professor Owen and Mr. Clark,[11] and Dr. Vernon.[12]

---

[1] Otto, in his Pathological Anatomy, (South's translation, pp. 269, 270,) refers to cases in which, in imperfectly formed fœtuses, the heart has consisted only of an expanded vascular trunk, or a single valveless cavity.

[2] Miscellanea Curiosa, Méd. Phys., sive Eph. Med. Phys. Germ., annus quartus et quintus anni 1673–74, Francofurti et Lipsiæ, 1676, obs. 40, p. 37.

[3] Ibid., Norimbergæ, 1691, obs. 44, p. 79.

[4] Phil. Trans., vol. 88, 1798, p. 346.

[5] On Malformations of the Human Heart, 1814, p. 2.

[6] Path. Trans., vol. 1, 1846–47, 1847–48, p. 48.　　　　[7] P. 228.

[8] Arch. Gén. de Méd., tom. 19, p. 257, quoted from Philadelphia Journal of Med. and Phys. Sc., vol. 14, 1827 ; N. S., vol. 5, p. 253.

[9] Arch. Gén. de Méd, 3me, et Nouvelle Serie, t. 15, 1842, p. 316.

[10] Path. Trans., vol. 1, 1846–47, 1847–48, p. 49.

[11] Lancet, 1848, vol. 2, p. 664.　　[12] Med.-Chir. Trans., vol. 39, 1856, p. 300.

The subject of the case recorded by Mr. Wilson was a child born at the full period, and which lived seven days. Though occasionally livid, it was generally pale, and died of slough-ing of the parietes of a sac which contained the heart, and which, owing to a considerable defect in the tendinous portion of the diaphragm, and to the absence of the lower part of the pericardium, formed a tumour projecting from below the sternum to the middle of the abdomen. Within this sac the heart rested upon the convex surface of the liver. The organ consisted of a single auricle and ventricle, and gave off a vessel which, after furnishing the pulmonary branches, proceeded upwards posteriorly to the thymus gland, behind the sternum, and then divided into the usual aortic branches. The thymus gland was unusually large, the pulmonary artery was much smaller than the aorta, and there was no ductus arteriosus.

In Dr. Farre's case, the child at birth was of full size, and though it breathed with some difficulty, and was slightly livid, it subsequently, for forty-eight hours, seemed to enjoy perfect health. "His countenance was lively and ruddy, his skin warm, and he took the breast eagerly." His breathing then became difficult and remarkably quick, the heart beat strongly, and his cries expressed distress. The skin became pallid and cold, the pulse at the wrist could not be felt, and he died seventy-nine hours after birth. On examination, the heart consisted of only one auricle, ventricle, and artery. The venæ cavæ opened into the auricle, and the pulmonary veins into the appendix, which was more distinctly separated from the sinus than usual. There was only one ostium ventriculi, and the ventricle gave origin to a single vessel, which furnished first the two pulmonary branches, and then the usual systemic arteries, together with a vessel which passed down to the heart, and formed the coronary arteries.

The case of Mr. Forster was very similar to the last. There was only one auricle, which received the two cavæ and two pulmonary veins, and opened into a ventricle from which a single vessel originated. This artery gave off two pulmonary branches, and the coronary arteries were derived from a trunk which apparently arose from the concavity of the aortic arch.

The subject of the case was a male infant, to all appearance well developed ; it however refused the breast, and had several attacks of dyspnœa, in one of which it died seventy-eight hours after birth.

In each of these cases the condition of the heart was very rudimentary, and the peculiar origin of the coronary arteries would appear to indicate that the division of the bulbus arteriosus had not taken place. In the following cases the heart had attained a higher state of development.

In the case which occurred in the practice of Mr. C. Clark, and is described by Professor Owen, the heart consisted of three cavities, two auricles, with distinct auricular appendages, and one ventricle ; but the left auriculo-ventricular aperture was obliterated, so that the left auricle communicated with the common ventricle only through the medium of the foramen ovale and the right auricle. The ventricle gave origin to a single artery, and the coronary arteries arose by a common trunk from the right subclavian artery. The child in which this malformation was found was puny and livid when born, but acquired a more natural colour afterwards. It again became livid, and died convulsed on the third day.

The subject of Dr. Vernon's case was a robust male infant, which appeared healthy at the time of birth, but its breathing was difficult and the surface discoloured, on the second day, and it died in convulsions, on the third day. On examination, the right auricle was found of large size, and was separated from a rudimentary left auricle only by a fleshy column and the fold of the valve. The left auricle received two pulmonary veins, but had no direct communication with the ventricle. The right auricle opened into a ventricle which was without any division, and gave origin to a single vessel. This vessel first gave off two pulmonary arteries, and then divided into the arteria innominata and the left carotid and subclavian arteries. The coronary arteries were derived from a common trunk which proceeded from the innominate artery.

The case related by Mr. Standert in the Philosophical Transactions, occurred in the practice of Dr. Combe, and the preparation, which is contained in the collection of Dr.

Ramsbotham, was exhibited at the Pathological Society in 1846, and is re-described in the first volume of the Transactions.[1] Through the kindness of Dr. Ramsbotham, I have had the opportunity of examining this specimen. There are two distinct auricular appendages, and the division of the cavity is indicated by a muscular band in the usual situation of the septum. The ventricle is large, and of a somewhat quadrangular form, and gives origin to the aorta, from which the coronary arteries arise as usual. There is another cavity forming a cul-de-sac in front of the aortic orifice, which is partially separated from the larger ventricle, and is evidently the analogue of the right ventricle, though it does not present any rudiment of a pulmonary artery. From the published account it appears that the pulmonary circulation was supplied from the aorta through the ductus arteriosus ; but that vessel is not retained in the preparation. We are informed that the child from which the heart was removed lived ten days, and was very livid throughout its life, though the functions of respiration and nutrition appeared to be otherwise naturally performed.

The cases of M. Mauran, M. Thore, and Dr. Crisp, afford examples of still more advanced development. In the first of these the auricle was provided with two distinct auricular appendages. The cavæ entered on the right side of the common cavity, and the pulmonary veins, which were only two in number, on the left. The auricle opened into an undivided ventricle, by an aperture guarded by a valve having the tricuspid form. The ventricle gave origin to the aorta, and also to a rudimentary pulmonary artery which was obliterated at its commencement. The trunk of the latter vessel, however, was pervious, and the pulmonary branches had received a supply of blood from the aorta, through a largely-open ductus arteriosus. In this case the child, which was a female, at the time of birth was small, but appeared healthy. When moved, it had attacks of difficulty of breathing in which it became livid, and uttered cries of distress, and it died in one of these when ten and a half months old.

In 1842, M. Thore described the case of a female infant

[1] Page 48.

which he saw at the Hospice des Enfans Trouvés, which presented general cyanosis, and had attacks of dyspnœa, with rapid breathing, a dry cough, and slight convulsions. It died when somewhat more than four months old. The heart consisted of only two cavities—an auricle and a ventricle ; the former was nearly spherical, and appears to have had two imperfectly developed appendages; it received the systemic and pulmonic veins, and opened into the ventricle by a single aperture. The ventricle gave origin both to the aorta and pulmonary artery; but the latter vessel was much the smaller of the two. The ductus arteriosus did not exist.

The case of Dr. Crisp was that of a child which had the usual symptoms of blue disease, and which died convulsed when ten weeks old. The preparation is retained by Dr. Crisp, and I have been favoured by that gentleman with the opportunity of examining it. The heart affords a good example of the transition from a single to a double set of cavities. There are two auricles, of which the sinus and appendix of the right are of large size, while the left auricle is rudimentary, and the inter-auricular septum is very imperfect. The auricles receive the usual veins, and open by a common aperture into a large ventricular cavity— the right ventricle —which is in connection with a rudimentary, but impervious, pulmonary artery. From the upper and right side of this cavity there is a communication with a second smaller sac—the representative of the left ventricle, from which the aorta takes its origin. The aorta doubtless furnished the supply of blood to the pulmonary branches and lungs through the ductus arteriosus; but that vessel has been cut away in making the preparation.[1]

From the description which has been given of these cases, it will be evident that they afford examples of hearts in very different stages of development. The cases of Mr. Wilson, Dr. Farre, and Mr. Forster, presented the simple biloculate condition of the organ ; while those related by Mr. Clark and Professor Owen, Dr. Vernon, Mr. Standert and Dr. Combe, Mr. Mauran,

---

[1] A case very similar to some of those which have been quoted, is referred to by Dr. Chevers, as seen in an infant which lived nine days, by M. F. Tiedemann.

M. Thore, and Dr. Crisp, illustrate the gradual advancement from the simple form of the heart to that in which it consists of four cavities. The cases of Mr. Clark and Professor Owen and Dr. Vernon are more closely allied to the former class of malformations; the others more nearly approximate to that which is next to be described.

HEART CONSISTING OF THREE CAVITIES.

In this description of malformation, the process of development is not arrested till a later period of fœtal life than in the class of cases last named, and the organ is found to have attained a more advanced condition. Thus, the auricular sinuses are separated by a more or less complete septum, and there are generally two auriculo-ventricular apertures; while the ventricle is either wholly undivided or presents only a very rudimentary septum. The arteries which are given off are usually two in number,—an aorta and pulmonary artery. This kind of defect, though very rare, is of more frequent occurrence than the biloculate heart. A case, which appears to have been of this description, was described by Chemineau, in 1699 ;[1] one was related by Tiedemann, in 1808-10 :[2] a specimen exhibiting a similar state was shown to Dr. Farre by Mr. Lawrence, in 1814,[3] and cases have been described by Fleischmann in 1815,[4] by Hein in 1816,[5] by Kreyzig[6] and Wolf in 1817, and more recently by Breschet,[7] Thore,[8] and Hale.[9]

In the case of Chemineau, the child had apparently only just breathed, and the heart is stated to have had three ventricles from the third of which the aorta and pulmonary artery arose.

Tiedemann's patient, who had suffered from the usual symptoms of morbus cæruleus, lived to the age of eleven, and the

---

[1] Hist. de l'Acad. des. Sc., p. 37.   [2] Zoologie, t. 1, p. 177.
[3] Malformations, p. 30.   [4] Meckel. Arch. f. d. Phys., 1815, p. 284.
[5] De istis cordis deformationibus quæ sanguinem venosam cum arterioso misceri permittunt.—Gœttingæ, 1816, p. 37.
[6] Krankheiten des Herzens, vol. 3, p. 200.
[7] Sur l'Ectopie, etc., obs. 1.
[8] Arch. Gén. de Méd., t. 1, 4mo serie, 1843, p. 199.
[9] Path. Trans., vol. 4, 1852-53, p. 87.

heart was found to have two auricles and one ventricle, and from the latter cavity the aorta and pulmonary artery arose.

In the specimen which was shown to Dr. Farre by Mr. Lawrence, the venæ cavæ and pulmonary veins opened as usual into their respective auricles ; but the inter-auricular septum was very imperfect, consisting only of a small muscular band, which left a large foramen ovale without any valve ; the septum ventriculorum was altogether wanting, and the ventricles communicated with the auricles by a common aperture. The aorta and pulmonary artery arose from the left side of the ventricle, and the orifice of the latter vessel was somewhat contracted. The history of the child was not known ; but, from the size of the heart, it was inferred to have lived some months.

The case of Fleischmann differed in some degree from these, as, though the heart consisted of three cavities, the ventricle only gave origin to one vessel, the orifice of the pulmonary artery being impervious. The child had lived twenty-one weeks. Hein's patient was a young man, who had been livid, and had suffered from difficulty of breathing and other symptoms of malformation, from early life, and who died of an abscess in the lung when sixteen years of age. There were two auricles, but the fold of the foramen ovale was perforated in three places. The auricles led by distinct apertures into a ventricle which had only the vestige of a septum, in the form of a membranous fold extending from the apex on the posterior side. The aorta and pulmonary artery arose from the common ventricle, and the latter vessel was of small size, and its valves converted into a ring. The ductus arteriosus was closed.

The case described by Kreyzig, is one which occurred to Mr. Wolf, and the heart is preserved in the Berlin Museum. It consists of two well-formed auricles, with distinct auriculo-ventricular apertures. There is an opening in the valve of the foramen ovale, and only one ventricle, from which two arteries arise. The valves of the pulmonary artery are imperfect. The subject of the malformation was a young man twenty-three years of age.

In the Archives Générales de Médécine for 1828,[1] a case is quoted from Hufeland's Journal, which occurred to M.

---

[1] T. 18, 6ᵐᵉ année, 1828, p. 83.

C

Wittcke, in a man twenty-four years of age, who had been subject to violent palpitation from infancy. He was attacked with peripneumony, followed by aggravated difficulty of breathing, amounting ultimately to orthopnœa; dropsical symptoms set in, and he died exhausted. The pericardium was adherent to the heart everywhere except at the apex, where it was wanting. The heart was very greatly enlarged, and the walls of the ventricle fully three times their usual thickness: there was not a trace of the inter-ventricular septum, but the positions of the vessels of the heart were natural, and the orifices were somewhat dilated. A volume of the same journal for the previous year,[1] contains a case quoted from a German publication, which may have been similar to this, but it is very imperfectly reported. The patient had always been delicate and livid, and had suffered from spitting of blood, palpitation, and dyspnœa, and he died of marasmus when thirty-five years old. It is stated that there was no inter-ventricular septum; but in this there seems some mistake, as the cavity of the right ventricle is reported to have been almost obliterated by the thickening of its parietes.

M. Breschet, in 1826, described the heart of a child which he had examined with M. J. F. Meckel of Halle, and which presented this form of malformation. The child was a male and was born at the full period, did not present any peculiarity of colour, and lived a month. In addition to other imperfections, a spina bifida, &c., the heart was situated on the right side of the chest. The right auricle was very large, and had two openings by which it communicated with the left auricle. There were two descending venæ cavæ, and the pulmonary veins opened into the right auricle. The ventricle was undivided, and gave origin to a large aorta which passed to the right side of the spine. The pulmonary artery was imperforate at its orifice, and its branches received blood from the ductus arteriosus.

In 1853, Dr. Hale exhibited to the Pathological Society the heart of a male infant, which, when born, was healthy-looking and well formed, but had afterwards occasional attacks of vomiting, with difficulty of breathing coming on in paroxysms. While quiet, the surface was warm; but during the attacks, the

---

[1] T 15, 5me année 1827, p. 110

extremities became cold. When seen by Dr. Hale, ten weeks after its birth, the surface of the body, the lips and hands, were pale, but had the natural tint. The pulsations of the heart were tumultuous and strong, and the pulse full and rapid. There was a superficial whizzing sound, heard at the sternum near the third cartilage. The child survived nine weeks longer, and was found dead in bed. The heart was much enlarged. The auricles were dilated, the appendices much increased in size, and the lining membrane thickened. The foramen ovale was wide and open, and the valve-like fold thicker than usual. The tricuspid orifice and valves were natural, but the mitral orifice was large and patulous. The ventricle was without the slightest rudiment of a septum. The aorta and pulmonary artery arose in their ordinary positions : the former was about double its natural size ; the latter, by comparison, being much smaller than usual. The semilunar valves of the pulmonary artery were large, thickened and irregular, but apparently competent ; the aortic valves were natural. The ductus arteriosus probably existed, though it did not occupy its usual situation.

The cases which have just been quoted, corresponded so far as that the heart consisted of two auricles and only one ventricle; but in other respects they differed in some degree. Thus, in the cases of Fleischmann and M. Breschet, the common ventricle gave origin to only one vessel—the aorta ; while the pulmonary artery, though it existed, was impervious at its orifice, and its branches received the blood, which they transmitted to the lungs, from the aorta through the ductus arteriosus. In all the other cases, on the contrary, there were two distinct vessels given off from the common ventricle. In the case of Mr. Lawrence, also, there was only one auriculo-ventricular aperture; whereas, in the other cases, two distinct openings existed.

In some cases which are on record, the heart has been found to present this form of malformation, combined however with irregularity in the origin of the large vessels. M. Breschet[1] has described the case of a male infant, whose heart was exhibited at the Société Anatomique,[2] by M. Martin. The child was

---

[1] Sur l'Ectopie, obs. 2ᵐᵒ p. 9.　　　　[2] Bulletin, 1ʳᵉ année, 1826, p. 39.

born at the full period, and lived six weeks, suffering during that time from dyspnœa, vomiting and convulsions. It was cold but not apparently cyanosed. The heart was situated in the median line, with its apex slightly inclined to the left side; it was of natural size, and had only one auricle, but with distinct auricular appendages; and there were two ascending and two descending cavæ. The aorta and pulmonary artery arose from the common ventricle, but their points of origin were transposed. There were two communicating arteries in the place of the ductus arteriosus;—one of which united the brachio-cephalic trunk and the right branch of the pulmonary artery; the other passed from the left pulmonary branch to the aorta.

A heart, displaying defects in some respects similar to those in the last case, has been described by M. Thore.[1] There were two distinct auricular appendages, but the cavities of the auricles freely communicated. The ventricle also presented the rudiments of a septum, but there was only one auriculo-ventricular aperture, and the points of origin of the aorta and pulmonary artery were transposed. The infant which was the subject of the malformation lived eleven days. It had a dry, hard, cough; and dyspnœa, increased on drinking liquids; but it was not cyanotic.

In the Museum of St. Thomas's Hospital there is a preparation which also affords an example of this condition. The specimen has no history attached to it; but, from the size of the heart, it was probably removed from a child eight or ten years of age. There are two auricles; but the right auriculo-ventricular aperture is obliterated, so that the blood from the right cavity must have flowed through a largely open foramen ovale, into the left auricle, and thence into the ventricle. The auriculo-ventricular valve rather resembles the mitral than the tricuspid valve. The ventricle is a single cavity, but presents a rudimentary septum, in the form of a thick fleshy column extending down its posterior wall, and the two arteries to which it gives origin, are transposed;—the aorta arising in front, in the usual situation of the pulmonary artery, while the latter vessel pro-

[1] Arch. Gén. de Méd., 4me serie, t. 1, 1843, p. 199.

ceeds from the posterior part of the ventricle. Cases of this description are closely allied to those hereafter to be described, in which, with transposition of the vessels, the septum of the ventricles is defective, and they only differ from them in the extent of the septal imperfection.

HEART CONSISTING OF FOUR CAVITIES ;—ONE OR BOTH OF THE SEPTA IMPERFECT.

When the partition of the ventricles is incomplete, the arrest of development may be almost entire, so that, as in some of the cases last mentioned, there may be merely a muscular band projecting into the cavity; or the deficiency may be very slight, one or more small apertures only existing at the upper part of the septum.

When the inter-ventricular septum is only partially defective, the imperfection most generally occurs at the base, where, during fœtal life, the division of the cavities is last effected. In this situation there naturally exists in the fully developed organ, a triangular space, in which the ventricles are only separated by the endocardium and fibrous tissue on the left side, and by the lining membrane and a thin layer of muscular substance on the right. This space indicates the point at which, in the turtle, there is a permanent communication between the two aortic ventricles; and it is interposed in man between the base of the left and the sinus of the right ventricle. Laterally it is bounded by the attachments of the right and posterior aortic valves, and its base is formed by the muscular substance of the septum. The dimensions of the space vary with the size of the heart; but ordinarily in the adult, the sides may be estimated at about seven lines, and the base is somewhat wider. When the lower part of the space is perforated, the left ventricle and origin of the aorta communicate with the sinus of the right ventricle; but, if the defect be situated high up, towards the angle of attachment of the valves, the communication may be between the left ventricle and the right auricle.

Generally when an aperture occurs in this situation, or, as it has been termed, in the *undefended space*, it has a triangular form; but, in some cases, it is oval or rounded; and in others, there are two or three apertures. When there is no source of obstruction at the right side, so that the right and left ventricles retain their just proportions and the flow of blood is from the left to the right side, the openings from the left ventricle are usually larger than those into the right ventricle. Not unfrequently, also, under such circumstances, as the apertures enter the right ventricle immediately below the ring of the auriculo-ventricular opening, the folds of the tricuspid valve become expanded by the column of blood flowing into the right ventricle, so as to form one or more small sacs. This has been pointed out by Dr. Thurnam[1] as shown in a specimen in the Museum of the Royal College of Surgeons, and probably the sac was thus formed in a case described by Dr. Pereira,[2] as one of partial aneurism of the heart.

While, however, deficiencies in the septum cordis are most commonly situated at the base, they are not confined to that situation. Occasionally, though, so far as my observation serves me, very rarely, the division between the left ventricle and the infundibular portion of the right, is perforated, so as to form a communication between the left ventricle and the origin of the pulmonary artery. In some cases, also, openings occur nearer the apex; and in yet others, several openings are found in different parts of the septum.

The defects in the inter-ventricular septum which have been enumerated, may co-exist with imperfect separation of the cavities of the auricles; but such is not always the case; and, on the other hand, the auricular septum may be imperfect or the foramen ovale unclosed, while the partition of the ventricles is entire. When also the auricular cavities are imperfectly divided, the septum may be scarcely developed, and the valve entirely absent; or the septum and valve may both exist, but only in a rudimentary form; or the septum of the auricles may be fully formed, but the valve may be very imperfect, so as to be incapable of covering the opening; or the orifice may be entirely

1 On Aneurisms of the Heart.—Med.-Chir. Trans., vol. 21, 1838.
2 Lond. Med. Gaz., 1845.

closed by the valve, and an aperture may exist in some other part of the auricular partition.

Occasionally the imperfection exists at the base of the heart, where the septa of the auricles and ventricles should unite, and thus a peculiar form of malformation results, in which the four cavities communicate. A case of this kind has been described by M. Thibert,[1] which occurred in a man who lived to the age of twenty-four, and presented no signs of disease of the heart till six weeks before his death. A similar preparation was some time ago sent to me by Dr. Curtis, now of Alton, which had been removed from the body of a girl, about twelve years old, of whose previous history no satisfactory account could be obtained. In this case the free communication between the left ventricle and the right ventricle and auricle, had been prevented by the expansion of a portion of the curtain of the tricuspid valve in the manner just described.[2]

It has been contended by some writers, and especially by M. Bouilland, that the apertures which are found in the septum ventriculorum are not always congenital; and there can be no doubt that perforations of the septum do occasionally, though I believe rarely, take place as the result of disease in after life. I have myself met with two cases in which disease existed at the undefended space at the base of the left ventricle,[3] which would have led to perforation, had life been prolonged; and a specimen of a similar description was exhibited at one of the earlier meetings of the Pathological Society, by the late Mr. Avery. A case is also related by M. Corvisart,[4] in which the writer is doubtful whether the perforation was not due to disease. I cannot, however, agree with M. Bouilland in regarding all the instances which he has quoted, as affording examples of communications so produced; and it is probable that some other cases, reported by more recent writers as the results of disease,

---

[1] Journal Gén. de Méd. 2me serie, t. 8, 1819, p. 254.

[2] Path. Trans., vol. 1, 1846–47, 1847–48, p. 61.

[3] Path. Trans., vol. 2, 1848–49, 1849–50., p. 49. See also notices of perforations supposed to depend on disease, by Dr. Bennett, in vol. 1, p. 59 ; and by Dr. Wilks, in vol. 6, p. 103.

[4] Mal. du Cœur, 3me ed. 1818, p. 287.

have been congenital defects. Generally there can be but little difficulty in deciding as to the congenital or accidental origin of the apertures in any given instance; for, in a large proportion of cases, the existence of other irregularities will afford unmistakeable evidence; and, in others, the triangular or rounded form of the openings and their smooth and polished edges, will indicate their nature. It must also be borne in mind, that when the edges of the openings are rough and irregular from fibrinous deposits, affording evidences of endocarditis, this does not alone show that the apertures are the result of disease; for such changes constantly accompany defects, unquestionably of congenital origin.

Deficiencies in the partitions of the auricles and ventricles usually co-exist with other important deviations from the natural form and development of the heart, and especially with some source of obstruction at the pulmonic or other orifice. But even large apertures are occasionally found in one or other of the septa, in persons who have died of affections unconnected with the heart who had presented during life no signs of obstruction or disorder of the circulatory system, and in whom the organ is otherwise well formed and free from disease.

In the Museum of St. Thomas's Hospital there are specimens which illustrate several of these forms of defective development. In No. 572, there is a small aperture in the undefended space of the left ventricle, by which that cavity communicates with the sinus of the right ventricle. This specimen was removed from a man, twenty-three years of age, who died of phthisis, and does not appear to have presented any signs of cardiac lesion. No. 1435A is a preparation of the heart of a child, six years of age, who presented no signs of disease of the heart till ten weeks before death, when she had scarlet fever. When admitted into the hospital, two weeks after the commencement of her illness, she had palpitation and a systolic bruit was heard over the whole chest, but loudest in the left axilla. She died of bronchitis and œdema of the lungs, and there were no indications of cyanosis. An opening, nearly circular in form and six lines in diameter, exists at the upper part of the septum atriorum, above the foramen ovale, and the latter passage is closed, except that a small valvular communication still exists. No. 1438 exhibits a deficiency in the septum cordis of a young person. The aperture is of considerable size, and the aorta, which is unusually large, arises above it, so as to communicate with both ventricles. The mouth of the pulmonary artery is not contracted.

Nos. 1435 and 1436 afford examples of the rare form of defect in which communications exist between the left ventricle and the infundibular portion of the right ventricle; but, as in these specimens there are other remarkable anomalies, I shall allude to them more fully hereafter.

A specimen in which a communication existed between the left ventricle and right auricle, was exhibited by Mr. Daldy to the Hunterian Medical Society, in 1853, which I have been favoured by Mr. Hilton with the opportunity of examining.

In the first plate,[1] I have given a representation of deficiency in the inter-ventricular septum, from a specimen exhibited at the Pathological Society, by Dr. Quain, in 1856. The preparation was taken from a youth, eighteen years of age, who died of phthisis, at the Brompton Hospital, under the care of Dr. Cursham. He had been cyanotic since he was two years of age. The "aperture was sufficiently large to permit a florin to pass through," and was remarkable for occupying the whole of the undefended space, and for its regular triangular form. The other drawing,[2] in the same plate, represents the usual situation of the opening into the sinus of the right ventricle, and is taken from a specimen exhibited by myself at the society, in 1849, and of which the preparation is retained in the Museum of the Hospital for Diseases of the Chest, Victoria Park. It was removed from a patient, whose case will be hereafter detailed, who had presented the usual aspect of morbus cæruleus, and died when seventeen months old.

---

[1] Plate 1, fig. 1.
[2] Plate 1, fig. 2.   The preparation is marked B 11 in the Museum.

1.—*Defect in the Interventricular Septum ; Pulmonary Artery arising directly or indirectly from the left Ventricle.*

In one of the most interesting forms of malformation the septum of the ventricles is not only incomplete, but is found to deviate from its natural position, one of the ventricles being unduly developed, while the other is atrophied. If this deviation of the septum be to the left side, the right ventricle is of large size ; and, while the pulmonary artery retains its natural position, the aorta also may arise wholly or in part from the same cavity. If, on the contrary, the deviation be to the right, both the aorta and pulmonary artery may originate from the left ventricle, and that cavity will be unduly developed. The former condition is of frequent occurrence, but the latter is rarely seen. A case which was related to the Académie des Sciences by M. Mery, in 1700,[1] was, however, probably of this description ; though it has been quoted as an example of biloculate heart. The fœtus was of very defective conformation, the large cavities being open. The heart consisted of a common auricle, into which both the pulmonary veins and the venæ cavæ entered. This cavity communicated by a considerable aperture with the right ventricle, and by a smaller one with the left ventricle. The right ventricle had no artery arising from it, but opened into the left, which gave origin both to the aorta and pulmonary artery.

A case occurred to M. Maréchale,[2] which affords an example of this kind of defect. Both the pulmonary artery and aorta arose from the left ventricle, and that cavity was of large size ; while the right ventricle was rudimentary, and communicated with the right auricle and the left ventricle. The auricular cavities were imperfectly separated. The subject of the case was an infant, which attained the age of nearly four

---

[1] Hist. de l'Acad. des Sc. année 1700, Paris, 1703, obs. 17, p. 42.

[2] Quoted in Gintrac, sur la Cyanose, (obs. 46, p. 173) from the Jour. Général de Méd., 1819.

months, and presented the usual symptoms of malformation of the heart.

A case related by Mr. Holmes,[1] of Montreal, also presents a somewhat similar malformation. It occurred in a young man, who died at the age of twenty-one, after having, throughout his life, laboured under palpitation, dyspnœa, and blueness of the lips, terminating in dropsical symptoms. The two auricles both opened into the left ventricle, and the right ventricle had no connection with the right auricle, but gave origin to the pulmonary artery, and communicated with the left ventricle by an aperture in the septum. Since this case was published, another, resembling it in several respects, has been recorded by M.Valleix.[2] The subject of the malformation was an infant which had double hare-lip, and died when about eight days old, after having undergone the operation. During its short life it presented no evidences of defect of the circulatory organs. The viscera of the body generally were transposed. There were two auricular appendages, but only a common cavity. Into this cavity two descending cavæ opened, one on the right, the other on the left side. The inferior cava entered on the left side, and the pulmonary veins on the right. The auricle opened into a large left ventricle by an aperture guarded by a tricuspid valve. The left ventricle gave origin to the aorta, and communicated with a second cavity, which was as it were hollowed out of the ventricular walls, and represented the right ventricle. This cavity gave origin to the pulmonary artery, and had no communication with the auricle, except through the other ventricle. The ductus arteriosus was natural.

[1] Ed. Med.-Chir. Trans., vol. 1, 1824, p. 252.
[2] Bullet. de la Soc. Anat., année 9, 10, 1834-35, p. 253.

2.—Defect in the Inter-ventricular Septum; Aorta arising in part from the right Ventricle; obstruction at the Pulmonic Orifice.

When the septum deviates to the left, so that the aorta acquires a communication with the right ventricle, there is most generally some source of obstruction at or near the origin, or in the course, of the pulmonary artery. The first case of this kind which appears to have been reported, is one which fell under the notice of Sandifort,[1] and was published in 1777. The subject of the case was a boy, twelve and a half years old, who had experienced great difficulty of breathing and palpitation of the heart, and had been unusually livid since he was a year old. The pulmonary orifice, owing to the adhesion of its valves, was so contracted as only to admit the passage of a small probe. The septum of the ventricles was imperfect, so that the aorta arose in part from the right side, and the foramen ovale was also open. In 1783 Mr. Hunter reported a case which he had occasionally seen for several years,[2] and which proved fatal in 1761. The boy was always dark-coloured, and had presented the usual symptoms of malformation of the heart since shortly after birth, and was remarkably thin. He was liable to paroxysms of difficulty of breathing, but could arrest them by lying down on the carpet when they were coming on. There is some uncertainty as to the age to which this patient survived: in the paper he is stated to have been thirteen years old, but, in the description of the plate, he is said to have been only eleven. On examination, the orifice of the pulmonary artery was found very greatly contracted, and the septum of the ventricles was imperfect, as in the case of Sandifort; but the foramen ovale, though not expressly mentioned, may be inferred to have been closed. In 1785 a third case of the kind was published by Dr. Pulteney,[3] which had occurred in 1781, and appears to have been communicated to the College of

[1] Obs. Anat. Pathol. cap. 1, § 10, 1782.
[2] Med. Obs. and Enq., vol. 6, 1783, p. 299, case 2.
[3] Med. Trans. of College of Phys., vol. 3, 1785, p. 339.

Physicians before the publication of Dr. Hunter's paper. The patient was a boy who died of acute dysentery at the age of thirteen years and nine months. The symptoms which he presented were similar to those in the two former cases, and he was especially remarkable for the darkness of his face and hands, and his liability to faintness on exertion. The period at which these symptoms first appeared is not mentioned. The ring of the pulmonary artery was much smaller and firmer than usual; and the septum of the ventricles was defective, so that the end of the finger could be passed from the aorta into either ventricle. The foramen ovale was most probably closed. In 1793, Mr. Abernethy[1] related an example of this form of malformation, in which, however, the child died when only two years old. The symptoms, as in the case of Dr. Hunter, appeared shortly after birth. The pulmonary artery was of small size; the aorta arose from the right ventricle; the septum cordis was imperfect, and the foramen ovale was largely opened. In 1795, the history of a similar case was communicated to Dr. Duncan[2] by Dr. Nevin of Downpatrick. The child which was the subject of the malformation presented no peculiarity till nearly two months after birth; it then had oppression of the chest, difficulty of breathing, and lividity. The symptoms became more marked when it was four months old, and it died at the age of ten months. The aorta at its commencement was large, and it was connected equally with both ventricles. The pulmonary valves were adherent together and ossified at their bases, and the artery was contracted. The foramen ovale would admit a large probe, but the ductus arteriosus was impervious. The case occurred at Glasgow, and the specimen is said by Mr. Burns to be contained in Dr. Jeffreys' Museum. Since the publication of these cases many others have been described in this country, France, Germany, Italy, and the United States. Indeed, as remarked by Dr. Farre, of the various deviations from the natural conformation of the heart, defects of this kind are the most common.

[1] Med. and Surg. Rev., vol. 1, 1795, p. 25; and Surg. Essays, 1793, vol. 2, p. 157.

[2] Duncan's Medical Commentaries, Edinburgh, vol. 19, 1795, p. 325.

Generally, in cases of this description, the number of the pulmonic valves is defective, and they are otherwise diseased; but there may be constriction of the orifice itself, or of the pulmonary artery. When the number of the valves is defective, there may be only two segments ; or the orifice may be imperfectly closed by a membrane stretched across and perforated in the centre ; or the valvular apparatus may be still more imperfect, being only represented by a duplicature of the lining membrane, or by a band of muscular fibres surrounding the orifice.[1]

When only two valves exist, one of the curtains is generally much larger than the other, and presents evidences that it originally consisted of two distinct segments, which have become united together ; the former line of separation being indicated by a ridge or frenum, extending from the edge of the valve to the side of the artery. When the valvular apparatus has the form of a perforated membrane, or, as it has been termed, of a diaphragm, the three segments are united together, and there are three ridges or frena, on the upper side, with corresponding sulci or furrows, on the ventricular side.

Whatever be the form of the valvular apparatus, the curtains are generally protruded forwards in the course of the artery; so as to give the opening from the ventricle a funnel shape, and to form deep sinuses between the valves and the sides of the vessel. The orifice itself varies in shape according to the number of segments. When there are two distinct valves, it is generally in the form of a slit, extending from side to side : when on the contrary, there is only a perforated membrane, the opening is usually triangular or rounded. In some cases the bases, as well as the free edges of the valves, are contracted, and the orifice has a tubular or barrel shape.[2] Occasionally the constriction is not caused by disease of the valves, but is

[1] Crampton : Trans. of College of Phys. of Dublin, N. S. vol. 1, 1830, p. 34 ; and Cyclop. of Anat. and Phys. vol. 2, p. 634. Favell : Prov. Med. and Surg. Jour., vol. 3, 1842, p. 440.

[2] These different forms of valvular disease are figured in plate 1, fig. 3 ; plate 2, figs. 2, 3, 4 ; plate 3, figs. 1, 2 ; plate 4, fig. 1; and also in figs 1, 2, and 3, plate 7.

situated at the outlet of the ventricle ; and depends on disease of the fibrous zone to which the valves are attached, or on hypertrophy of the adjacent muscular substance and thickening of the endocardium.[1] Obstruction may also be caused by general smallness of the pulmonary artery ; and by rigidity of the orifice, which prevents its expanding duly with the progress of growth.

The size of the orifice varies greatly in different cases. It may admit the point of one of the fingers, or a lead pencil, or common quill ; or it may only allow of the passage of a crow-quill or probe. M. Louis has recorded a case in which, in a man twenty-five years of age, it measured only two and a half lines in diameter; and M. Bertin found the aperture to have the same size in a female of fifty-seven. I have myself measured the capacity of the orifice in two males, fifteen and twenty years, and in a female nineteen years of age, and found the circumference thirteen, twelve, and eight French lines respectively :— the average size in adults being about thirty-six French lines. In two children, six and a half and two and a half years of age, the circumference of the orifice was six and a half and five French lines.

In most cases the valves are not only adherent but they are otherwise much diseased, being thickened, irregular, and indurated ; and, if life be sufficiently prolonged, not unfrequently contain larger or smaller masses of cretaceous deposit. From the similarity of these changes to those which result from inflammation in after life, they may be referred to that process occurring during fœtal existence. Generally, also, the valves become the seat of subsequent disease and display recent deposits or vegetations, by which the contracted opening is often still further diminished in size. In most cases, at least when all the segments are united together, the valves are incapable of entirely closing the aperture.

The trunk of the pulmonary artery is in some cases dilated, in others it is smaller than usual ; and its coats may either be thickened and indurated, or they may be thin and transparent, more resembling those of veins.

[1] This condition is represented in plate 4, fig. 2.

In most cases of this description of malformation, the foramen ovale does not become entirely closed ; but such is not always the case, the septum of the auricle being in some instances entirely imperforate ; while in others the foramen ovale may close naturally, but an aperture may exist in some other portion of the auricular partition. The ductus arteriosus occasionally remains pervious ; and the tricuspid valves are frequently diseased, the folds being adherent at their edges, and their surfaces studded with fibrinous deposits or vegetations.

With an imperfectly divided ventricle, the heart may possess its natural form externally, and the defect may only be detected on laying open the cavity ; but more generally, and especially when the septal defect is considerable, the organ is wider than usual, resembling the quadrangular form of the heart of the turtle. This change is more marked when, with deficiency in the inter-ventricular septum, there is some obstruction to the exit of the blood from the right ventricle, by the pulmonary artery. The infundibular portion of the right ventricle is then usually imperfectly developed, its cavity very small and the walls hypertrophied ; while the sinus is much enlarged, its parietes acquire a greatly increased width and are peculiarly tense and resisting. and the muscular columns become much hypertrophied. In a boy of ten, and a girl of nineteen years of age, the walls of the right ventricle measured 5 and $5\frac{1}{2}$ French lines in thickness ; —the average width in adults, of the two sexes, being 1·93 and 1·87 French lines.[1] The right auricle undergoes great dilatation, and its parietes become unusually thick. The left cavities on the contrary are, relatively, much smaller, and their walls thinner and more flaccid.

While, however, the chief valvular disease, and the most marked hypertrophy and dilatation, are found in the right cavities of the heart, the changes are not entirely limited to that side, but affect, to a less degree, the left also. Thus the folds of the mitral valve are not unfrequently found opaque and thickened, and the

[1] See Papers on the Weight and Dimensions of the Heart in Health and Disease, by the author, in the London and Edinburgh Monthly Journal of Medical Science for 1854.

aortic valves may be in a similar condition, or the number of the curtains may be irregular. The hypertrophy and dilatation of the left ventricle are most marked in persons who survive for some years; and, in such cases, the general enlargement of the heart and the increase of weight which it attains, are often considerable. In the two patients before referred to, the organ weighed 10 oz. and 17½ oz. avoirdupois respectively, though the normal weight, at the same ages, should not exceed eight or eight and a half ounces.

Some discussion has arisen as to the cause to which the hypertrophy of the right ventricle in cases of malformation is to be ascribed; and it has been supposed by Bertin, Bouilland, and others, to be due to the entrance of aërated blood, through the aperture in the septum. This explanation cannot, however, be accepted as satisfactory. When there exists any source of obstruction at the right side of the heart, as in by far the majority of instances in which the septum is imperfect, the course of the blood through the aperture will be from the right ventricle into the left; and it is probably only in the comparatively small proportion of cases, in which, with a defective septum, there is no source of obstruction on the right side, that the reverse obtains. In the latter class of cases, however, the right ventricle does not become hypertrophied to any great extent, though the patient may survive for many years. But, whenever there exists any source of obstruction at or near the pulmonic orifice, and whenever the deficiency in the septum is so great as to throw upon the right ventricle a large share in the maintenance of the systemic circulation, the right ventricle is invariably found more or less hypertrophied; even though the life of the patient may be prolonged only for a few weeks or months. The ventricular parietes also acquire as great an increase in width and firmness, in the cases in which there is obstruction at or near the pulmonic orifice without any defect in the inter-ventricular septum, and therefore without any entrance of aërated blood, as when that partition is imperfect. It seems therefore evident, that the hypertrophy of the right ventricle in these cases, is due to causes precisely similar to those which occasion hypertrophy of either ventricle in after life;—the increased growth which is consequent on the powerful muscular efforts to overcome the obstruction occasioned by the contracted or rigid state of the pulmonic orifice, or to maintain the circulation in the systemic, as well as in the pulmonic vessels.

It has been thought that in cases of malformation, the right ventricle sometimes presents what has been termed true "*concentric hypertrophy.*" It is now admitted, that, in accordance with the observations of Cruveilhier and Dr. Budd, in ordinary cases of hypertrophy, the cavity affected either retains its natural dimensions or undergoes dilatation; and that diminution of capacity is only observed when an unusually powerful ventricle has been violently contracted at the period of death, as in some instances of rapidly fatal hæmorrhage.[1] The exception to this rule, supposed to be afforded by cases of malformation, is, however, most probably, only apparent. I have several times examined imperfectly developed hearts, in which the right ventricle has been very small when the organ was first removed from the body; but, after they have been macerated till the muscular tension is relaxed, the cavity uniformly expands to a larger size, and the thickness of the walls undergoes a proportionate diminution. Specimens exhibiting very thick parietes with small ventricular cavities, are, indeed, to be found in museums; but they have probably been placed in spirit before the muscular contraction has subsided, and thus the temporary state has been retained. The term concentric hypertrophy has also been applied to the condition of a ventricle from which the blood has been diverted into other channels, in consequence of which the cavity has become much reduced in size, and the parietes proportionately thicker. The term is, however, still less applicable to this condition which is one of atrophy, not of hypertrophy.

In speaking of imperfection in the inter-ventricular septum, it has been mentioned that the defect may exist in very different degrees. The extent to which the septum may be misplaced may also vary greatly. In some cases only a small portion of the aortic orifice, as one-third or one-fourth of its circumference, is in connection with the right ventricle. In others, the aorta

---

[1] See case by author, in Path. Trans., vol. 1, 1846-47, 1847-48, p. 85.

is placed immediately above the incomplete septum, so as to communicate equally with both ventricles; and, in yet other instances, it arises wholly from the right ventricle. An example of the latter condition was exhibited at the Pathological Society, in 1846, by Mr. Ward and Dr. Parker.[1] The heart had been removed from the body of a boy, who died of pneumonia, at the age of thirteen, and had been cyanotic from birth. The valves of the pulmonary artery were united so as to form a diaphragm, with an aperture in the centre which would only admit a small quill. The ascending aorta, as is always the case when that vessel communicates freely with the right ventricle, was of large size. The left ventricle formed only a small supplementary sac, opening from the right ventricle; and the latter cavity was unusually large, and its walls thick.

In the museum of St. Thomas's Hospital there are various specimens exhibiting deficiency in the inter-ventricular septum, with obstruction at the pulmonic orifice. No. 1440 is a preparation of this kind, removed from the body of a child twelve months old, which had suffered from dyspnœa from birth, and had been livid and subject to frequent convulsive attacks. The pulmonary artery is of small size, and is provided with only two valves. The septum of the ventricles is imperfect, so that the aorta is in communication with the right ventricle. The inter-auricular septum is also very defective; the left auricle imperfectly developed; and there are two superior venæ cavæ. No. 1437 is a similar specimen, except that the pulmonary valves are united together, so as to form an infundibular or funnel-shaped opening from the ventricle into the artery. The preparation was probably obtained from a subject nine or ten years of age, but has no history attached to it.[2] In No. 1439 the pulmonary orifice is much contracted, owing to the adhesion of the two valves with which it is provided, so as to leave only a circular aperture. The septum ventriculorum is defective, and the aorta arises above the aperture, and communicates with both ventricles. The foramen ovale and the ductus arteriosus are

---

[1] Path. Trans , vol 1, p. 51.

[2] The form of the pulmonic valvular apparatus in this case is displayed in plate 4, fig. 1.

both closed. The preparation was formerly in the museum of Sir Astley Cooper. It was removed from a boy, nine years and five months old, the particulars of whose case, accompanied by a drawing of the heart, are given by Dr. Farre.[1] At the time of birth nothing unusual was observed in his appearance; but, a few months after, his complexion became dark; and, at the age of two and a half, his lips and cheeks had a bluish-black colour, which was heightened by passions of the mind and by cold. From this period till his death he was always similarly affected, not only by mental causes, but also by slight corporeal exertion, particularly in very cold weather, and his extremities were cool to the touch. Before he was three years old he lost the use of the lower extremities, but recovered under the care of Dr. Babington. He complained of nausea and headache from the earliest period at which he was able to express his feelings. Shortly before his death he was seen by Sir Astley Cooper and Mr. Wheelwright. He died of abscess in the right hemisphere of the brain, with hemiplegia and convulsions. This case is further remarkable as presenting a contraction of the infundibular portion of the right ventricle, anterior to the orifice of the pulmonary artery—a condition which will hereafter be alluded to.

In my own practice I have met with several instances of this description of malformation.

CASE I.[2]—*Great Contraction of the Orifice of the Pulmonary Artery; Aorta arising chiefly from the right Ventricle; Foramen Ovale and Ductus Arteriosus closed.*

The boy who was the subject of this malformation first fell under my notice in June, 1846. He was then two years and one month old. I was informed that he was born healthy, and continued to thrive till he was vaccinated at the age of three months. Shortly after this he began to decline in health, and

---

[1] Malformations, p. 24. The case of John Cannon.

[2] Path. Trans. vol. 1, p. 52, and Edin. Monthly Jour. of Med. Sc., vol. 7, 1847, (or N. S., vol. 1), p. 644. The preparation of the heart in this case is contained in the Museum of the Victoria Park Hospital, and is numbered B4 in the Catalogue. It is represented in figs. 1 and 2, plate 2.

gradually became worse, till, when six months old, he was much in the same state as when brought to me.

His mother had previously had two other children, both of whom were remarkably healthy. While pregnant with this child, and two months before her confinement, she was frightened by seeing a child killed, and never recovered the shock she sustained.

When first seen, the child's face was tumid, the cheeks of a deep rose colour, and the lips livid. The sternum was arched and prominent, and the ribs flattened above and expanded below. The abdomen was tumid, and the body generally emaciated. The hands and feet felt cold, and the fingers and toes were of a deep blue colour, and their extremities enlarged and club-shaped, more especially the thumbs and great toes. The super-ficial veins in different parts of the body were very conspicuous. Several of the teeth were decayed, the mucous membrane of the mouth and tongue was in an unhealthy state, and the angles of the lips were ulcerated. There was also a livid excoriation around the anus. The pulse was extremely quick (136), and feeble and irritable. The cartilages of the ribs in the præcordia were prominent, and the dull space was increased in extent. A loud blowing, and somewhat rough murmur, accompanying the impulse of the heart, was heard over the whole præcordia, and along the course of the sternum, on each side of the lower part of that bone, and in the epigastrium. It was perceived also in the neck and in the dorsal region on the left side of the spine. It was, however, most intense and rough in its character at the inner side of, and immediately above, the left nipple. The murmur was succeeded by a distinct second sound, but of a duller or flatter character than usual.

The child was of very irritable disposition, and, when unduly excited or fatigued by exertion, was subject to paroxysms of extreme difficulty of breathing, attended with violent palpitation of the heart; lividity, almost amounting to blackness, of the face, hands, and feet; and general turgescence of the super-ficial venous trunks.

For about two months, the child was occasionally brought to me, and I afterwards lost sight of him till the 5th of October.

I then found him much weaker than before ; his head was large, and his mother thought had latterly much increased in size. He was greatly emaciated, and his appetite was extremely defective; his face pale ; lips, hands and feet livid; and the superficial veins, especially those of the neck, very large. The extremities were cold, and the fingers and toes more clubbed than before. The abdomen was tumid, and the mouth and anus still ulcerated. The præcordia yielded a dull sound from the third intercostal space to the edges of the ribs, and from the left of the sternum to the line of the nipple. The cartilages of the fourth, fifth and sixth ribs, were especially prominent. From the extreme irritability of the child, it was impossible accurately to investigate the physical signs; but the loud systolic murmur was heard very distinctly on the inner side of the nipple, and along the course of the sternum. The action of the heart was extremely rapid. On the evening of the day on which these notes were taken he was seized with convulsions, at first confined to the upper extremities, but subsequently becoming general. He continued sensible at intervals till the 7th, when he became comatose, and he died at two o'clock in the afternoon of the following day. During the last few hours he had violent palpitation of the heart, great lividity of the face and extremities, and extreme dyspnœa. He was two years and five months old at the time of his death.

The body was examined at noon on the 9th. The head was large and the anterior fontanelle somewhat open; much fluid was effused in the subarachnoid cellular tissue and into the ventricles. At the base of the brain a layer of soft and recently exuded lymph extended from the optic commissure to the posterior part of the pons Varolii, and passed for a considerable distance on each side, more especially in the course of the Sylvian arteries, so as to envelope the nerves proceeding from this part of the brain. In some places, the deposit was fully two lines in depth. The subjacent cerebral substance, as also the parts contained in the ventricles, presented no appearances of disease. The brain weighed 37 oz. avoirdupois. The liver extended from the level of the fifth rib above, to an inch and a-half below the edges of the cartilages, and across the entire upper part of the abdomen. It weighed 14 oz., and was of a deep purple colour, and very solid. The spleen was large and firm; the kidneys labulated and congested; and the stomach and intestines healthy. Several small hæmorrhoidal excrescences were found around the anus, and the epithelium was there abraded.

The lungs were sparingly crepitant; the bronchial glands large, and the thymus also still of large size. The heart occupied its usual site; it was large for the age of the subject, and broader in its transverse than in its longitudinal axis. It measured in girth $5\frac{1}{2}$ French inches. The right ventricle occupied almost the entire front of the organ, and the great firmness of its walls presented a striking contrast to the softness and flaccidity of those of the left ventricle. The right cavities were distended with blood of a dark colour and tarry consistence. The right and left venæ innominatæ, the vena azygos and the cavæ, were unusually capacious. The right auricle was much larger than the left, and its walls averaged nearly a line in thickness. The Eustachian valve was two or three lines in width, and the lining membrane of the auricle was opaque. The foramen ovale was entirely closed by its valve, and the fold formed a deep sac projecting into the left auricle. The right auriculo-ventricular aperture admitted a cylinder two inches and eleven lines in circumference. The valves were thickened, but apparently competent to close the orifice. The right ventricle was unusually capacious, and its walls were thick, measuring near the base $2\frac{1}{2}$ French lines, at the midpoint 4 lines, and near the apex $2\frac{1}{2}$ lines. The columnæ carneæ were large and firm. The infundibular extremity of the ventricle admitted a ball measuring one inch in circumference; but the orifice of the pulmonary artery was contracted to a mere slit, two lines in length, situated between two valves, which were of a firm and fleshy character, and protruded forwards into the cavity of the artery. The trunk of the artery, though of very small calibre, was, in reference to the orifice, disproportionately large, and its coats were unusually thin. At the usual point it divided into three branches, two of which were distributed to the lungs; and the third—the ductus arteriosus—though at first pervious, became entirely obliterated towards its union with the coats of the aorta.

A strong muscular band crossed the upper part of the
ventricle, eight lines below the origin of the pulmonary artery,
and in front of the auriculo-ventricular aperture, so as partially
to divide the cavity into two portions; the anterior of which
gave origin to the pulmonary artery; while that situated
posteriorly opened directly into the aorta, by an orifice allow-
ing the passage of a cylinder one inch and nine lines in
circumference.

The pulmonary veins entered the left auricle as usual. The
left auriculo-ventricular aperture was smaller than the right,
measuring only one inch and ten lines in circumference; the
valves were natural. The cavity of the left ventricle was
relatively smaller, and its walls thinner, than those of the left,
measuring $2\frac{1}{2}$, 3, and 2 lines in width. The columnæ carneæ
were small and flaccid. The opening from the left ventricle into
the aorta was indirect, and smaller than the communication
between that vessel and the right ventricle. There could
scarcely be said to be any deficiency in the inter-ventricular
septum, though, through the aorta, the two cavities communicated. There were three semilunar valves at the orifice
of the aorta, two of which corresponded with the right, and
one with the left ventricle; the valves were natural. The
ascending portion of the aorta was very large; it gave off the
usual branches at its arch, and below the attachment of the
impervious ductus arteriosus it diminished to about its natural
calibre. The bronchial arteries were scarcely traceable, and the
intercostal branches had their natural size.

This case affords a good example of the form of malformation
in which the pulmonic orifice is obstructed and the septum of
the ventricles imperfect. It differs, however, from the majority
of such cases, in having had the foramen ovale closed and the
septum of the auricles entire; and this, notwithstanding that
the contraction of the pulmonic orifice was very marked.

The following case affords an instance of the more common
variety of this malformation, in which the foramen ovale is
open. For the particulars of the case I am indebted to Mr.
Marshall, of Mitcham, in whose practice it occurred.

CASE II.[1]—*Deficiency in the Septum Ventriculorum; great Contraction of the Pulmonary Orifice; open Foramen Ovale; Ductus Arteriosus closed.*

" G. S., aged six years and a half, was born at the full period; was rather dark coloured, and did not run alone till he was twenty months old. His mother stated that, at the fifth month of her pregnancy, she was much frightened. When the child was three years and a half old, he had a fit, and was paralysed on the right side. The face soon recovered; but the arm and leg were ever after weak, particularly the former. As the child has increased in size, so have his symptoms become more severe. His breathing has become shorter, so as to be hurried on the slightest exertion, and the surface has acquired a deeper tinge. My first acquaintance with the case occurred two years before the boy's death, when he was brought to me suffering from extreme dyspnœa, even when at rest, which was unusual with him. His condition at that time was as follows:—

" Skin of a purple hue, eyes large and appearing to start from the orbits, conjunctivæ slightly injected, extremities very purple, nails almost black, and ends of fingers much flattened. The chest was narrow and prominent in front. The action of the heart was tumultuous and forcible, and the sounds confused; the respiration was quickened. A few days before his death he took measles, and had passed mildly through the disease, when he was seized with convulsions, occurring every few minutes, and terminating in coma, with dilated pupils, and the eyelids half open. The fæces and urine were passed involuntarily, and the surface of the body was darker than usual, and the conjunctivæ highly congested. The boy died on the evening of July 31, 1853, and the body was inspected thirteen hours after death.

" The head was not examined, but all the organs of the chest

[1] Path. Trans., vol. 5, 1853–54, p. 67. The preparation of this case is preserved in the Museum of the Victoria Park Hospital, and is numbered B 6 in the Catalogue. The form of the pulmonic orifice is represented in plate 2, figs. 3 and 4.

and abdomen, except the heart, were found healthy, though much congested."

The heart, which was sent to me by Mr. Mitchell, was of large size, and, the right ventricle especially, was hypertrophied and dilated. The pulmonary orifice was so greatly contracted, owing to the adhesion of the valves, that a cylinder of six and a half French lines in circumference could only be introduced into the vessel. The valves were united into a hollow cylinder attached to the coats of the vessel on one side, but elsewhere separated from them by a deep sinus; the passage from the ventricle into the vessel being thus three or four lines long. The trunk of the artery also was of small size. The septum of the ventricles was deficient at the base, over a large space, so that the aorta arose from both ventricles. The opening from the right ventricle into the aorta, had a capacity of twenty-one French lines; that from the left ventricle into the vessel, of twenty-four lines. The foramen ovale was so freely open as to admit of the passage of the forefinger. The ductus arteriosus was closed.

In the following case the foramen ovale was closed, as in the first which I have related, but the ductus arteriosus was still pervious.

CASE III.[1]—*Contraction of the Orifice of the Pulmonary Artery; Imperfection of the Septem Ventriculorum ; Foramen Ovale closed ; Ductus Arteriosus pervious.*

R. B., a female, aged nineteen, was admitted into St. Thomas's Hospital in July, 1854. She was born at the full period, but from birth was of a peculiarly dark colour. When ten months old she began to suffer from violent fits of crying and excitement, in which she became black in the face; and these fits sometimes terminated in convulsions. The paroxysms recurred at intervals of a few hours or days, till she was five years old, when they ceased; but she continued subject to transient attacks

[1] Path. Trans., vol. 7, 1855–56, p. 80. This preparation is numbered B 7 in the Catalogue of the Museum of the Victoria Park Hospital. The form of the pulmonic orifice is represented in plate 4, fig. 2, and the situation of the open duct, in plate 5, fig. 1.

of vertigo and headache. About the same time she had sores on the limbs, for which she was sent to Brighton. After the cessation of the paroxysms she continued much in the same state till she was fourteen or fifteen years of age. She still suffered from palpitation and dyspnœa, aggravated by mental excitement or by corporeal exertion, and her health then became more impaired. When she was eighteen years of age, the catamænia appeared for the first time, and she had only three or four imperfect recurrences afterwards. She now became subject to frequent catarrhal attacks, and had, on several occasions, spat large quantities of blood, and had bled freely from the nose.

Her mother stated that when she was pregnant with this child, and four or five months before her confinement, she was greatly alarmed by her husband, who was insane, standing over her for two hours with a loaded pistol.

When she was admitted into St. Thomas's in July, she presented the usual symptoms of malformation of the heart, with signs of obstruction at the right side, and marked cyanosis. Her cheeks were livid, and the colour did not quickly return into them when they were blanched by compression. The conjunctivæ were injected; and the lips, gums, and interior of the mouth were of a dark purple hue, and the gums spongy and tender. The nails were much arched and dark-coloured, and the extremities of the fingers were somewhat bulbous. The chest was prominent in front, and flat at the sides. There was very obvious pulsation in the carotids, and the jugulars were distended, but did not pulsate. She suffered from great difficulty of breathing and sense of suffocation, and was often incapable of lying down in bed. Her extremities were cold, and she felt constantly chilly; the pulse was quick (120); the beat of the heart was ill-pronounced, but of tolerable power. Her appetite and digestion were good, but the dyspnœa and palpitation were increased after taking food. The præcordial dulness commenced at the level of the third cartilage, and continued to the edges of the ribs. Laterally it extended from the left side of the sternum to fully an inch beyond the left nipple. On listening over the third cartilage, between the nipple and sternum, a soft blowing murmur was heard very distinctly. It was audible, though less intensely, over the whole præcordia, and in a line towards the middle of the left clavicle. It was also distinctly heard to the right of the upper part of the sternum. A loud ringing second sound was heard, about the middle and at the upper part of the sternum, after the murmur. A very marked thrill was felt on pressing the intercostal spaces, over the whole præcordia, but especially between the third and fourth cartilages. The heart's sounds were heard in the left dorsal region, but the murmur was not there audible. The chest was sparingly resonant on both sides, and respiration was harsh, but unattended by rhonchus.

While in the hospital she did not improve, and she was discharged at her own desire. She was again admitted, after an absence of a month, at the end of August, when the cholera was prevailing, and was then much worse; the lower extremities, which were before somewhat swollen, were very œdematous, and the abdomen also was tumid, and the general symptoms and physical signs were much as before. Soon after her re-admission she was seized with bilious vomiting, the bowels being at the time confined. She was relieved by treatment, and, after two days, when she had apparently recovered her ordinary state, she was suddenly attacked with diarrhœa of the usual choleraic character, and rapidly sank into fatal collapse.

On examination, the brain, lungs, liver, spleen and kidneys, were found greatly congested, but not otherwise diseased. The intestines contained the gruel-like fluid which is commonly met with after death in the second stage of cholera. The heart was very greatly enlarged, weighing 17½ oz. avoirdupois. The right auricle was distended with uncoagulated blood, and was greatly dilated, and its walls hypertrophied, measuring two to three French lines in thickness. The foramen ovale was closed, the fold being drawn up above the isthmus and entirely adherent; the valve was somewhat thickened. The tricuspid valves were opaque and thick, and studded with wartlike vegetations on their auricular side.

The right ventricle formed nearly the whole of the anterior portion of the heart; its cavity was much enlarged, and its walls firm and resistant, and very thick, measuring from three to seven lines in width in different parts. It had two openings; one of large size, from the sinus into the aorta; the other very small from the infundibular portion into the pulmonary artery. This aperture was so greatly constricted as only to admit of the passage of a cylinder having a circumference of eight French lines. The constriction was situated at the bases of the valves, and was formed by a muscular band covered by fibrous tissue, and the edges of the opening were studded with warty vegetations. Immediately beyond the constriction the passage expanded, so that the valves themselves freely admitted the forefinger between them.

The segments were two in number, and one of them displayed some remains of a frenum or band on the upper surface. Except being somewhat thickened and opaque, they were free from disease. There was a deep sinus behind each of them. The pulmonary artery was of small size, but very much larger than the orifice.

The left auricle was small, and its walls averaged one line and a half in thickness. The mitral aperture and valves were healthy. The left ventricle was less capacious and its walls thinner and much less firm than those of the right; in width they ranged from two to six French lines.

The aorta arose much to the right of the pulmonary artery, and communicated with the sinus of the right ventricle by an aperture thirty-three French lines in circumference, and with the base of the left ventricle by an opening thirty-six French lines in circumference. The aortic valves were natural. The ascending portion of the aorta was of large size, but the vessel diminished considerably after giving off the vessels to the head and upper extremities. The ductus arteriosus was pervious, and sufficiently large to give free passage to a crow-quill.

In 1849, I exhibited at the Pathological Society[1] the heart of a child seventeen months old, which presented similar malformations to those in the last case. The child had been under the care of Dr. Oldham, and had presented the usual symptoms of morbus cæruleus. It died of effusion on the brain, preceded by icterus. The heart was very large for the age of the child; the pulmonary orifice was of small capacity, and was provided

[1] Path. Trans. vol. 2, 1848-49, 1849-50, p. 37. The preparation is marked B 11 in the Museum of the Victoria Park Hospital, and is represented in plate 1, figs. 2 and 3.

with only two semilunar valves; and there was an aperture at the base of the septum ventriculorum, sufficiently large to allow of the passage of the little finger. The aorta arose above the aperture in the septum, so as to communicate with both ventricles. The right ventricle and auricle were very large, and the walls of the ventricle were unusually strong and thick. The left cavities, on the contrary, were relatively small, and the parietes of the left ventricle were thinner and more yielding than those of the right. The foramen ovale was closed, except at its upper and anterior part, where there existed a valvular opening, which, when the auricle was distended, would have allowed of the passage of blood from the right into the left auricle. The ductus arteriosus was pervious, but would only admit of the passage of a very fine probe. The coronary artery arose at a point above its ordinary origin.

In the cases which have now been mentioned, the defective condition of the septum of the ventricles was associated with, and probably dependant on, the obstruction at the pulmonic orifice. Cases will hereafter be referred to in which the imperfection of the septum apparently depended on obstruction at the point of union of the infundibular portion and sinus of the right ventricle ; and, it is probable, that the septum may equally remain unclosed in consequence of disease of the right auriculo-ventricular aperture, and of the aortic or mitral orifices. In the *Lancet* for 1848, a case is related by Mr. Robinson,[1] in which the right auriculo-ventricular valves were diseased and the septum of the ventricles imperfect, in a child a year and a half old, without any defect at the pulmonic orifice. In a case recorded by M. Burguières,[2] the septum cordis was found imperfect in a girl of nineteen, in conjunction with some disease of the mitral valve and extensive obstruction at the aortic orifice, caused by the union of the valves into a diaphragm, leaving an aperture only fourteen lines in circumference.

In the following case, the defect in the inter-ventricular septum, co-existed with disease of the tricuspid valve.

---

[1] Vol. 2, p. 103.
[2] Thèses de la Faculté, Paris, 1841 ; quoted by Deguise, Thèse, 1843.

Case 3.[1]—*Two small Apertures in the Septum Ventriculorum; contraction of the right Auriculo-ventricular Aperture; Foramen Ovale and Ductus Arteriosus closed.*

A female infant was brought to me at the Hospital for Diseases of the Chest, on the 1st of March, 1853. It was then three months old, and was stated to suffer from paroxysms of difficulty of breathing, during which the face and upper extremities became very dark, and the heart beat violently. The child was unusually livid when born; but it subsequently acquired a more natural colour, and then again became darker at the end of the first week. The palpitation and dyspnœa were observed at the end of the second week; and those symptoms continued till she was brought to the hospital.

On the 2nd of March the following notes were taken:—"The child has had no severe paroxysm since she was last seen; but the hands and face have been constantly more or less livid; there is, however, now no blueness beneath the nails. The mother states that the left arm and hand are always of a darker hue than the right and that the limb is somewhat swollen, and such is certainly the case at present. The lower extremities are of the natural colour. The action of the heart is powerful, and there is a systolic murmur, audible over the whole front of the chest, but most intensely in the præcordia and to the left of the lower part of the sternum. It is also very distinct at the upper part of the sternum and beneath the left clavicle, but is less intense on the right side of the sternum. Behind, it is only indistinctly audible; but it is somewhat louder to the right than to the left of the spine. There is some dulness on percussion in the dorsal regions, especially the left. Bronchitic rhonchi are heard in all parts of the chest. The pulse is regular and equal at the wrists. The child is very restless and becomes extremely livid. when excited, as by crying, or even by the slightest exposure to cold." From this date the paroxysms were less frequent and severe, and the child had generally a more natural appearance ; but it did not thrive, or rather it became more emaciated.

In the beginning of June the child took hooping-cough, under which the other members of the family laboured at the time. The symptoms then became much aggravated; the breathing was rapid and laborious, and the action of the heart tumultuous. During the fits of coughing the face and extremities were intensely livid,—almost black,—and suffocation seemed impending. The child died convulsed on the 29th of June, when about seven months old.

The body was much emaciated. There were adhesions between the two layers of pericardium at the apex of the heart. The heart weighed 2½ oz. avoirdupois. Its form was somewhat more pointed than usual ; the apex was formed by the left ventricle. Both auricles contained coagula, and the left was very much distended by firmly coagulated but dark-coloured blood. The right auricle was of ordinary size ; the Eustachian valve distinct. The right ventricle was small, but its walls were thick and dense. The pulmonary artery was of unusually large size, its orifice admitting of the passage of a ball twenty-one French lines in circumference. The folds of the right auriculo-ventricular valve were thickened and adherent at their angles, so as to contract the dimensions of the orifice, which only admitted a ball measuring twenty-four lines in circumference. On the auricular surface of the valve there was a thick exudation of recent lymph. The cavity of the left auricle was large, and the walls thicker than usual. The foramen ovale was closed, but the fossa was depressed towards the left side. The left auriculo-ventricular aperture had a circumference of eighteen lines. The walls of the left ventricle were less firm than the right. The aorta arose from the left ventricle, but there were two openings in the septum ventriculorum, by which the ventricles communicated ; these apertures were much larger on the left than on the right side. Both openings led into the right ventricle, behind the auriculo ventricular valves, and the largest had a circumference of six lines. The ductus arteriosus was completely closed.

The glands at the root of the lungs and in the course of the large vessels were much enlarged. The thymus gland was large.

The lungs were in some places collapsed, in others emphysematous; much viscid mucus was contained in the smaller bronchial tubes in the collapsed portions of the lungs. The liver, spleen, and kidneys were engorged, but otherwise healthy.*

* In addition to the cases briefly noticed in the text, the following may be referred to.

Orifice of the Pulmonary Artery contracted, or the vessel small or rigid ; imperfection of the Ventricular Septum ; Foramen Ovale open.

Ring, Med. and Phys. Journal, vol. 13, 1805, p. 120. In a female child one year old. Gintrac, Sur la Cyanose, Paris, 1824, obs. 16e.

Duret and Calliot, Bullet. de la Fac. de Méd., 1807, p. 21. In a boy aged 11 years. Gintrac, obs. 20e ; Norman Chevers, M.D., Collection of Facts illustrative of Morbid Conditions of the Pulmonary Artery, (originally published in Lond. Med. Gaz., 1845–51) ; London, 1851, p. 27.

Obet and Calliot, Bullet. des Sc. Med., t. 2, 1808, p. 65 ; and Bull. de la Soc. de l'École de Méd., 1807, p. 24. In a male child 3 years old. Duct. art. pervious, but small. Gintrac, obs. 21e. Dr. Chevers, p. 25.

Huet, Bullet. de la Soc. de Méd., t. 2, 1808, p. 72. Aged 13 years. Hein ; De istis cordis deformationibus quæ sanguinem venosam cum arterioso misceri permittunt.—Gœttingæ, 1816, obs. 49e. Chevers, p. 32.

Palois, Bull. de la Fac. de Méd., t. 2, 1809. p. 133. In a male child 4½ years old. Gintrac, obs. 23e.

Knox, Ed. Med. and Surg. Jour., vol. 11, 1815, p. 57. In a female child four years old. Duct. art. absent. Gintrac, obs. 38e.

Ribes, Bullet. de la Fac. de Méd., t. 4, 1815, p. 422. In a male child, 6 years old. Gintrac, obs. 37e.

Haase, Diss. Inaug. Med. de Morbo Cœruleo, Lipsiæ, 1813, p. 7. Gintrac, obs. 26e. Hein, obs. 58. In a female who lived 9 years and 11 months. Duct. art. nearly impervious.

Travers, Farre on Malformations, 1814, case of H. B., p. 34. In a male who lived four years. Gintrac, obs. 35e.

Leadam, Ibid, p. 37. In a male who lived 22 years. Gintrac, obs. 36e.

Dorsay, New England Jour. of Med. and Surg., vol. 1, 1812, p. 69. Girl, age at death not stated ; but upwards of two years old.

Gintrac, Sur la Cyanose. obs. 45e, p. 164. In a man 21 years of age.

Cheevers, New England Jour. of Med. and Surg., vol. 10, or N.S., vol. 5, 1821, p. 217. In a male aged 13½ years. Duct. art. the size of a crow-quill.

Bloxham, Med. Gaz., vol. 15, 1835, p. 435. In a female aged 3 years.

Holst, Hufeland's Journal, 1837, quoted in Arch, Gén. de Méd., 2me serie, t. 11, 1836. p. 91. Dr. Chevers, p. 26. In a child 2 years old. The duct. art. opened into the left subclavian artery.

E

Tommasini, Clinica Medica di Bologna, quoted in Bouilland, sur les Maladies du Cœur, 2me ed. 1841, vol. 2, p. 674, obs. 183. In a female aged 25.

Lexis, Lancet, 1835-36, vol. 2, p. 483, with plate ; quoted from a German journal. Dr. Chevers, p. 28. In a female child 5¾ years old.

Napper, London Med. Gaz., vol. 27, 1841, p. 793. In a boy aged 5 years and 7 months old.

Hildenbrand, Arch. Gén. de Méd., 3me et nouv. serie, t. 14, 1842, p. 87. In a girl of 7 years. Left subclavian artery absent, and supplied by branches from the vertebral and left pulmonary arteries.

Landouzy, Ibid, 3me serie, t. 3, 1833, p. 436. Case of M. Magendie. In a female 8 years of age. Also Bullet. de la Soc. Anat., an. 13, 1838, p. 165.

Hope, Treatise on Diseases of the Heart, 3rd edition, 1839, p. 491. In a girl 8 years old.

Crampton, Trans. of the Dublin College of Physicians, N. S., vol 1, 1830, p. 34. In a boy, aged 11 years.

Iliff, Dr. Chevers' Collection, p. 34. In a female, aged 12 years.

Denucé, Bullet. de la Soc. Anat., an. 24, 1849, p. 124. In a female, aged 32 months.

Valette, Gaz. Méd. de Paris, 2me serie, t. 13, 1845, p. 97. Case under the care of M. Scouttetin. The preparation was shown to M. Sedillot, and is preserved in the museum at Strasburg. Female, lived 5 years. Chevers, p. 34.

Orifice of the Pulmonary Artery contracted, &c., imperfection of the Ventricular Septum ; state of the Foramen Ovale not reported.

Farre, Malformations, 1814, p. 24. Case of Sir A. Cooper and Mr. Wheelright. In a boy aged 9½ years.

Meyer, Hein, obs. 25, J. F. Meckel, Beitrag zur Geschichte der Bildungsfehler des Herzens welche die Bildung des rothen Blutes hindern.—Deutsches Archiv für die Physiologie.—Halle und Berlin, 1815, p. 221, obs. 42. In a female 7 years old.

Gregory, Med.-Chir. Trans., vol. 11, 1820, p. 296. In a boy aged 18 years. Gintrac, obs. 49^e.

Bertody and Dunglison, Phil. Med. Ex., 1845, quoted in Dublin Journal, vol. 28, 1845, p. 300. In a female 21 years of age.

Jackson, American Jour. of Med. Sc., vol. 43, 1849, p. 338. In a negro child aged 4 years.

Watson, Lectures, 2nd. ed., 1845, vol. 2, p. 247. In a male 17 years of age.

Pulmonary Orifice contracted, &c.; imperfection of the Ventricular Septum ; the Foramen Ovale closed.

Olivry, Journal Gén. de Méd., t. 73, 1820, 12me de la 2e serie, p. 145. In a male 6 years of age. Gintrac, obs, 47e.

Louis, Arch. Gén. de Méd., 2me serie, t. 3, 1823, obs. 9 ; and Mem. et Rech. Anatomico-Pathologiques, 1826, p. 313, obs. 10. In a man 25 years of age, combined with contraction of right auriculo-ventricular aperture.

Graves and Houston, Dublin Hospital Reports, vol. 5, 1830, p. 322, Case 1. In a boy, 3 years old. Duct. art. pervious, but narrow.

Blackmore, Ed. Med. and Surg. Jour., vol. 33, 1830, p. 268. In a girl, 3½ years of age. Great contraction, or possibly obliteration, of the left auriculo-ventricular aperture.

Marshall, Lond. Med. Gaz., vol. 6, 1830, p. 886. In a man 23 years of age.

Huss, Gaz. Méd. de Paris, t. 11, 1843, p. 91. In a boy 6 years old. No appearance of arterial duct. Chevers, p. 33.

Gravina, Schmidt's Jahrbücher, 1839, quoted in Arch. Gén. de Méd., 3me et nouv. serie, t. 6, 1839, p. 360. In a boy 9 years old. Chevers, p. 35.

Chevers, Collection of Facts, &c., p. 36. In a boy 16 years of age.

Chevers, Ibid. p. 36. In a person 15 or 16 years of age. Possibly with an open ductus arteriosus.

Escalier, Bullet. de la Soc. Anat., 20me an. 1845, p. 213. In a female, 11 years of age.

Dalrymple, Path. Trans., vol. 1, 1846-47, 1847-48, p. 58. In a female 25 years of age.

3. *Obliteration of the Pulmonary Orifice.*

A more aggravated degree of the kind of malformation to which allusion has just been made, is that in which the orifice or trunk of the pulmonary artery is entirely impervious. A case of this description was described by Dr. Hunter in 1783, in the paper before referred to.[1] The child was born at the eighth month, was very livid, had violent palpitation, and died in convulsions on the thirteenth day. The pulmonary artery was found entirely impervious and was contracted into a solid cord. The septum of the ventricles was entire, and the right ventricle had scarcely any cavity left, while the left ventricle was large and powerful. The foramen ovale continued open, and the pulmonary branches received their supply of blood from the aorta, through the medium of the arterial duct. In 1812, a specimen, similar so far as the obliteration of the pulmonary orifice is concerned, was briefly described in the London Medical Review; and in 1814, some further particulars of the same case, of which the preparation was in the possession of Mr. Hodgson, were given by Dr. Farre.[2] The pulmonary artery

[1] Med. Obs. and Enq. vol. 6, 1783, p. 291, case 1.
[2] London Med. Rev. vol. 5. 1812, p. 262 ; and Farre on Malformations, p. 19.

was reduced to an impervious filament leading to the ductus arteriosus. The latter vessel, which was of large size, was connected with the aorta, and gave off the pulmonary branches. In the septum of the ventricles "some of the muscular fibres were wanting, and the lining membrane of the left ventricle had three foramina, giving it a cribriform appearance." The foramen ovale was largely open, and the right auriculo-ventricular aperture and the corresponding ventricle were of small size. The left ventricle, on the contrary, was unusually large. The child was observed to be of a deep purple colour soon after birth, and had difficulty of breathing. It died in convulsions on the seventh day. In the same publication Dr. Farre[1] alluded to two other cases, which had occurred to Mr. Langstaff. One of these was that of a still-born child; in the other, the infant lived six months, and its temperature was always much below the natural standard; its skin of a deep colour, almost black; and it had fits daily. In this instance the septum of the ventricles presented a considerable perforation; but the opening and the cavity of the right ventricle generally, was almost filled up by muscular fibres. The ductus arteriosus was remarkably short, and very small. Dr. Farre mentions that he had examined a third specimen exhibiting this defect, and that a fourth had been mentioned to him. In 1816,[2] Mr. Howship published a case which agreed with that of Mr. Langstaff in the circumstance of the septum cordis being deficient; but the aorta arose above the aperture, and the right ventricle was unusually large and powerful, while the left cavities were of small size. The child, which first presented symptoms of cyanosis when fifteen days old, lived to the age of six months.

Since the publication of these cases, others of a similar description have been recorded both in this country and elsewhere, and specimens have been exhibited at the Pathological Society, by Drs. Crisp,[3] Chevers,[4] and Hare,[5] and I shall have again occasion

[1] On Malformations, &c., p. 27.
[2] Practical Observations in Surgery and Morbid Anatomy, 1816, p. 93.
[3] Path. Trans., vol. 1, 1846-47, 1847–48, p. 50.
[4] Ibid. p. 204.
Ibid. vol. 4, 1852-53, p. 81.

to refer to one shown there by myself. This kind of defect is, however, of much less frequent occurrence than that last described.

In some cases the obliteration is confined to the orifice of the pulmonary artery, and is caused by the union of the valves, forming a kind of septum or diaphragm, stretched across the opening, and entirely separating the cavity of the vessel from that of the ventricle, while the trunk of the artery remains pervious. In other instances a larger or smaller portion of the vessel, commencing at its origin from the ventricle and extending towards the ductus arteriosus, is impervious and converted into a ligamentous cord. When the whole of the trunk is obliterated, the pulmonary branches appear to be simply the divisions or continuations of the ductus arteriosus. Obliteration of the pulmonary artery, it will be seen from the short account which has been given of cases of this description, may occur at different periods of fœtal life; either in the early months, before the septum cordis is completely formed, or during the later periods, after the separation of the ventricles is entire. It is, however, of much the most frequent occurrence at the former period. Indeed, of twenty-four cases of this form of malformation of which I have collected notes, in four only, including that of Dr. Hunter, does the disease appear to have occurred when the septum of the ventricles was already completed. A fifth case of the same kind is referred to by Dr. Chevers as existing in the collection at Guy's Hospital. In most of the cases which have been described, the defect in the septum of the ventricles appears to have been considerable; but the preparation in the possession of Mr. Hodgson formed an exception to this rule.

If the obliteration occur while the growth of the septum is in progress, the right ventricle becomes large and powerful, and the aorta derives its chief supply of blood from that cavity, while the left auricle and ventricle are proportionately small. If, on the contrary, the obliteration occur after the septum of the ventricles is completed, the right ventricle and right auriculo-ventricular aperture become very much diminished in size, and the left cavities are unusually large and powerful. The latter condition also obtains when, as in the case of Mr. Hodgson, the communication between the ventricles is not free.

When the septum of the ventricles is imperfect, the foramen ovale is occasionally found closed. Thus there was no communication between the auricles in four out of the twenty cases referred to, and in two others the state of the foramen is not named in the reports. When, on the other hand, the septum of the ventricles is entire, the foramen ovale is necessarily pervious to some extent; though, as in a case exhibited at the Pathological Society by Dr. Hare, the opening may only be of small size.

Generally in cases of obliteration of the pulmonary artery, the lungs receive their supply of blood from the aorta, through the ductus arteriosus. Indeed, in twenty out of twenty-four cases, this seems to have been the channel through which the supply was obtained though it is not in every instance expressly stated. In one, however, of these cases, that related by M. Lediberder, the duct did not exist in its usual situation ; but there was an aperture in the trunk of the pulmonary artery, immediately below its bifurcation, by which it communicated directly with the aorta, and so the pulmonary branches obtained their supply. In two cases, however, the ductus arteriosus is reported to have been closed, and the sources of the pulmonary supply were not ascertained. In a third case, in which the duct was closed,— that of Dr. T. K. Chambers, as described by Dr. Chevers,[1]—the lungs received compensatory branches from the arch of the aorta ; and in that of Dr. Babington,[2]—also related by Dr. Chevers,—the supply furnished to the lungs through the ductus arteriosus was supplemented by the other vessels arising from the aorta. The blood circulating through the ductus arteriosus was distributed by two branches to the right lung, and by one very small and long vessel to the left lung. The left branch of the pulmonary artery was obstructed ; and the left lung received its supply partly through the small vessel, and partly through one of two additional branches which arose from the descending aorta. The other branch passed to the right lung. The period during which the patients survived in these instances was remarkable, both having lived to the age of nine or ten. In a case

[1] Collection of Facts, &c., p. 15.
[2] Ibid. p. 14. This preparation is marked 1383²⁵ in Guy's Hospital Museum.

related by Dr. Shearman,[1] however, in which the source of the pulmonary supply was not ascertained, the patient also lived to the age of nine ; and Dr. Crisp has related one in which the ductus arteriosus most probably conveyed the blood to the lungs, and the girl attained the age of twelve years.

A case, which is described as one of obliterated pulmonary artery is reported in the sixty-first volume of the Medical and Physical Journal,[2] and a preparation, which is probably that of the heart described, exists in the Museum of the London Hospital. By the kindness of my friend Mr. Nathaniel Ward, I have had the opportunity of examining this specimen, and find that it presents a condition, so far as I am aware, unique. The pulmonary artery is not obliterated, but exists as a vessel of very small size throughout its whole course. The aperture of communication with the ventricle is a mere slit in an opaque membrane stretched across the orifice, which will only admit the end of a small probe. This membrane is formed by the adhesion of the valves, which are apparently only two in number. The artery itself will admit a large crow-quill ; and it divides into the usual branches distributed to the lungs. There is no trace of the ductus arteriosus; but, about an inch below the origin of the left subclavian artery, a vessel arises from the aorta, the size of a goose-quill, which divides into two branches distributed to the left lung. About half an inch lower down a second but smaller vessel is given off, which is distributed to the right lung. The aorta is of large size, and is placed above a considerable aperture in the septum of the ventricles, so that it freely communicates with both cavities. The left coronary artery arises at a higher point than natural. The ventricles are both of large size. The foramen ovale is closed, but the Eustachian valve is fully developed. The specimen is stated in the catalogue to have been removed from the body of a female, sixteen years of age, who died of phthisis in the practice of Dr. Ramsbotham, and is doubtless that referred to in the Journal. The patient had during life presented the usual features of morbus cœruleus.

Cases of this description depend on the faulty development

---

[1] Prov. Med. and Surg. Journal, 1845. p. 484.   [2] P. 548.

of the branchial arches, by which the portions which form
the ductus arteriosus and pulmonary artery become obliterated,
to a greater or less extent, at an early period of fœtal life.
In all cases in which the pulmonary artery is completely
obstructed, while the ductus arteriosus remains pervious, that
vessel must necessarily become the channel through which the
blood is conveyed to the lungs. But if the portion of the
branchial arch which forms the ductus arteriosus becomes prematurely obliterated, the pulmonary artery will remain very
small, and may require other vessels to furnish a compensatory
supply; or, if the obliteration involve both the ductus arteriosus
and the pulmonary artery, the supply to the lungs may be
entirely derived from other sources. As the branches of the
bronchial arteries anastomine with those of the pulmonary
artery, they will furnish the most ready channel for this vica-
rious supply, and at an early period of fœtal life they are probably readily capable of undergoing the requisite dilatation.

The following case of obliteration of the pulmonary artery
has fallen under my own notice.

CASE IV.—*Obliteration of the trunk of the Pulmonary Artery;
Aorta arising chiefly from the right Ventricle and giving off
the Pulmonary Branches through the Ductus Arteriosus.*[1]

The subject of this case was a male child under the care of
Dr. Bentley, at the City Dispensary, in 1847, which I had
several times an opportunity of seeing and examining. His
mother stated that, at the time of birth, his skin was extremely
dark-coloured, but he breathed freely. The child was from the
first, restless and peevish; and, when three months old, began
to suffer occasionally from paroxysms of extreme excitement
and crying, during which his breathing became very rapid and
laborious; there was violent palpitation of the heart and of the
vessels of the neck and scalp, and great lividity of the face, with
convulsive contractions of the hands and feet.

[1] Pathological Transactions, vol. 1, 1846-47, 1847–48, p. 205. The preparation is contained in the Victoria Park Hospital Museum, and is marked
B 8. It is also delineated in plate 4, fig. 3.

When first seen by myself on November 15, 1847, the child was ten months old. He was then tolerably well nourished, and exhibited sufficiently characteristic, though not very marked, cyanosis. The lips were of a purplish colour, the lower eyelids dark, and the face pale and puffy. The extremities of the fingers and toes were somewhat bulbous, and the glandular portions of the finger and toe nails nearly black. The sternum was arched and prominent, and the lower ribs were much drawn in with the inspiratory act. There was some fulness, but no pulsation, of the jugular veins. A loud systolic murmur was audible over a large portion of the front of the chest, and less distinctly posteriorly, on the left side of the spine in the inter-scapular space; but the child was in so excited a state—crying continually and incapable of being quieted for a moment—that it was impossible accurately to investigate the physical signs. The head was of very unnatural form, being remarkably narrow and contracted anteriorly, and broad and elongated behind. The anterior fontanelle was closed, but the skull was very prominent in that situation.

The child continued to suffer from the attacks of dyspnœa which have been described, generally once daily, sometimes more frequently, according to the degree of severity and length of duration; a long interval existing between the paroxysms only when it had been completely exhausted. Towards the end of the seizures the breathing became quick and laborious, with a tendency to suffocation, and the face and extremities were extremely livid. The tongue was drawn up to the roof of the mouth, and the thumbs were pressed into the palm of the hand. The child refused the breast; and it died in one of these attacks, on the 11th of January, 1848, when wanting two weeks to being twelve months old. The father was a healthy man; but the mother was much out of health, and stated that, when pregnant with this child, she was greatly alarmed by seeing a man who was dying of asthma. They had but one other child, and that, though very healthy looking, was very backward for its age — between three and four years — being still incapable of speaking.

On the examination of the body, the integuments were found sufficiently provided with fat. The lungs were small, very much congested, and sparingly crepitant.

The pericardium was natural; the heart was of very large size for the subject, being much expanded transversely, and weighing $3\frac{1}{4}$ ounces avoirdupois. The right auricle was extremely large, and its walls unusually thick. The foramen ovale was covered by its valve, which, however, not being adherent to the isthmus, would allow the flow of blood from the distended right auricle into the left. The Eustachian valve was very imperfectly developed. The right auriculo-ventricular aperture and its walls were natural. The cavity of the right ventricle was of very large size, and consisted almost entirely of the sinus ; the infundibular portion was reduced to a mere chink, and was entirely closed at the usual point of origin of the pulmonary artery. The trunk of the pulmonary artery formed an impervious cord extending from the ventricle to the bifurcation of the vessel and its union with the ductus arteriosus. The septum of the ventricles was imperfect at the base. The walls of the right ventricle were extremely thick, measuring five to six Paris lines in width, and unusually firm. Relatively to the right cavities, the left auricle and ventricle were very small, and the walls of the latter were thinner and more flaccid. The valves were natural. The aorta arose in chief part from the right ventricle, and was of large capacity so far as the point at which it gave off a vessel, evidently the ductus arteriosus, through which the supply of blood had been transmitted to the lungs. This vessel communicated with the aorta at a point somewhat anterior to the natural situation of the duct, and was of sufficient size to admit a small goose-quill. After following a course of six lines, it divided into two branches transmitted to the right and left lungs, and from its point of bifurcation a small but solid cord, the impervious trunk of the pulmonary artery, passed down to the base of the right ventricle in the usual situation of the pulmonary artery. The coronary arteries and pulmonary veins were natural. The abdominal viscera were much engorged, and the parenchymatous organs enlarged and solid.

The case which has been related affords an example of oblite-ration of the pulmonary orifice occurring at the earlier period of fœtal life, before the septum of the ventricles is completed. Of the rarer description of cases in which the obliteration occurs after the division of the ventricles is effected, a specimen was exhibited at the Pathological Society by Dr. Hare in 1853.[1] It was removed from a male child, who was very livid, and died when nine months old. The right auricle was of large size, and the foramen ovale was open, but only to the extent of one-sixteenth of an inch in breadth, and one-tenth or one-twelfth of an inch in length. " On cutting into the right ventricle, it was found that the columnæ carneæ were fused almost into one," so that it presented nearly " a solid mass." The cavity would only hold a moderate-sized pea. The septum ventriculorum was perfect. The orifice of the pulmonary artery was entirely closed, but its trunk constituted a cul-de-sac in communication with the ductus arteriosus, and which divided into the usual branches. The orifice from the aorta would admit a crow-quill. The left ventricular walls were very thick, measuring fully half an inch, and the cavity gave, as usual, origin to the aorta.

The most interesting feature in the case was the extremely small size of the opening in the foramen ovale, considering that the passage afforded the only medium of communication between the right and left sides of the heart.[2]

[1] This specimen is preserved in the museum of University College, London.
[2] In addition to the cases of *obliteration of the orifice or trunk of the pul-monary artery* quoted above, the following may be referred to.

With the Septum of the Ventricles entire.

M. Lordat, Gintrac, obs. 53°. The child lived six weeks.

Dr. Carson, Ed. Med. and Surg. Jour., vol. 62, 1844, p. 134 ; and Dublin Jour., vol. 26, 1845, p. 126. In a child that lived 5 days.

With the Septum of the Ventricles imperfect.

Houston, Dublin Hospital Reports, vol. 5, 1830, p. 324, case 2nd. In a child which lived 18 months.

Fearn, Lancet, 1835, vol. 1, p. 312. ´In a child which lived 7 weeks. The ductus arteriosus is stated to have been closed, and the means by which the lungs were supplied with blood was not ascertained.

Spital, Edinburgh Med. and Surg. Jour., vol. 49, p. 109. In a child which lived 23 days.

Biggar, Quoted in Ed. Med. and Surg. Jour., vol. 55, p. 251, from German publication. The child lived 5½ months.

J. G. Smith, Lancet, vol. 1, 1841–42, p. 543. In a child which survived 8 months.

Douglas, Med. Gaz., vol. 31, 1843, p. 16. The boy lived 18 months.

Hall and Vrolik, quoted in Arch. Gén. de Méd., t. 8, 1828, p. 595. In a female child which lived 2 years.

Dr. Chevers, Path. Trans., vol. 1, 1846-47, 1847-48, p. 204. In a child apparently several weeks old, but without any history.

Dr. Crisp, Path. Trans., vol. 1, 1846-47, 1847-48, p. 50 ; and Diseases of Blood Vessels, p. 92. In a female, 12 years old.

Lediberder, Bullet. de la Soc. Anat., 11ᵐᵉ année, 1836, p. 68, in a boy 12 days old. The ductus arteriosus did not exist in its usual situation ; but a direct opening was found between the aorta and pulmonary artery.

Lawrence, Ibid, 12ᵐᵉ année, 1837, p. 216. In a female child which lived 15 days.

Shearman, Prov. Med. and Surg. Jour., 1845, p. 484. In a girl nine years of age. In this case the ductus arteriosus is stated to have been closed ; but the source of pulmonary supply was not ascertained.

SUPERNUMERARY SEPTUM IN THE RIGHT VENTRICLE.

Writers on cardiac pathology describe instances of duplicity of the cavities of the heart: thus Kerkring[1] states that he has seen the right ventricle double, with two pulmonary arteries. Probably, however, by far the majority of cases of apparent duplicity consist in the development of septa in the cavities, and it is thus that we may explain the remark of Andral,[2] that he has seen a heart with three auricles, and another with four ventricles. It is chiefly in the right ventricle that this irregularity is observed ; indeed that cavity is the only one in which I have myself ever seen a supernumerary septum developed.

The occurrence of this defect in the right ventricle has, I believe, been correctly ascribed by Mr. Grainger to irregularity in the development of the two portions of which the cavity originally consists. In the turtle, and other of the higher reptiles, the heart consists of three imperfectly separated ventricles ; the right and left systemic ventricles, from which the

[1] Dr. Paget on Congenital Malformations.—Edinburgh Med. and Surg. Jour., vol. 36, 1831, p. 289.

[2] Pathological Anatomy, translated by Townsend and West, vol. 2, p. 333.

two aortæ arise, and a small anterior ventricle which gives origin to the pulmonary artery. The latter is entirely separated from the left, but communicates with the right aortic ventricle. The sinus and infundibular portion of the right ventricle are, in man, the analogues of the right systemic and pulmonic ventricles of the turtle. The right ventricle in the well-formed human heart, always shows, at the point at which the two portions unite, some indications of division by the muscular columns to which the folds of the tricuspid valve are attached; and, in cases of malformation, this is still more marked. When also a supernumerary septum is developed, it is at the point of union of the sinus and infundibular portion that it occurs; and the partition of the cavity of the ventricle is by part due to hypertrophy of the muscular columns which usually occupy this situation, and partly to the thickening and induration of the lining membrane. The opening by which the portions of the ventricle communicate often consists of a firm fibro-cartilaginous ring, not unfrequently displaying old or recent deposits of lymph upon its edges. In form it is usually round or oval, and it may be so small as only to admit the passage of a crow or a goose-quill, or it may readily allow of the finger being passed through. The effects upon the general form of the ventricle vary with the degree of obstruction which the septum occasions, the sinus of the ventricle being large and thick, (and especially so when the septum cordis is also deficient, so that the aorta has a communication with the right ventricle), while the infundibular portion, (if there be no other source of obstruction at the orifice of the pulmonary artery), becomes atrophied, and is reduced to a very small cavity.

One of the earliest instances in which this condition of the heart appears to have been noticed, was in a specimen preserved in the museum of St. Bartholomew's Hospital, and described by Dr. Farre.[1] There does not appear to have been any history of the case; but the subject of the malformation was supposed to have been about fourteen years of age. The aorta arose from both ventricles, and the pulmonary artery was correctly formed and of natural size. A heart presenting a similar condition has been

---

[1] On Malformations, p. 26.

described and figured by Mr. Holmstead,[1] as found in a girl nine years of age ; and Dr. Crampton[2] has reported a third case which appears to have closely resembled the other two, except that the pulmonic orifice was destitute of valves, and was only closed by a puckering of the lining membrane, which occasioned some contraction.   The defect occurred in a boy ten years of age. Dr. Elliotson[3] has referred to a case probably of a similar kind ; and Dr. Theophilus Thompson[4] described another, in which the patient was a female 38 years of age, and the pulmonary orifice was wide and provided with four well-formed and equal-sized valves. A case has also been described by M. Chassinat,[5] in which there appears to have been a septum in the right ventricle, while the pulmonary orifice was entirely oblite-rated, and the branches to the lungs received blood through the ductus arteriosus. The malformation occurred, with other irre-gularities, in a child which lived twelve days. Examples of this defect have also been published by M. Aran and M. Deguise,[6] in a case which occurred in the practice of M. Honoré ; by M. Pize ;[7] and probably a case published in Hufeland's Journal,[8] may have been of a similar description. In 1847 Mr. Le Gros Clark exhibited, at the Medico-Chirurgical Society,[9] the heart of a young man, nineteen years of age, which presented this malformation He had laboured under symptoms of cardiac disease, with much lividity of the face, probably throughout his life. The orifice of the pulmonary artery was provided

---

[1] London Medical Repository, vol. 17, 1822, p. 455.

[2] Transactions of the College of Physicians of Dublin, N.S., vol. 1, 1830, p. 34, quoted in Todd's Cyclopædia of Anat. and Phys., vol. 2, p. 634.

[3] Lumleyan Lectures, 1830, p. 21.

[4] Med.-Chir. Trans., vol. 25, 1842, p. 247.

[5] Arch. Gén. de Méd, 2me serie, t. 11, 1836, p. 81.

[6] Lancet, 1844, vol. 1, p. 501 ; and Bullet. de la Soc. Anat., 17me année, 1842, p. 180, and Thèse de la Cyanose Cardiaque, &c. Paris, 1843. In a female 20 years of age who had suffered from the usual symptoms of malformation from birth.

[7] Thèse de la Fac. de Paris, 1854, No. 148, obs. 29, p. 31. In a man 22 years of age.

[8] Arch. Gén. de Méd., 2me serie, t. 2, p. 101, in a female of 25.

[9] Med.-Chir. Trans., vol. 30, 1847, p. 113.

with only two valves but it was not contracted, and immediately below the origin of the vessel there was a cavity of small size, partially separated from the other portion of the right ventricle; the only communication between the two cavities being through two small circular apertures, " neither of which would admit, without distension, the passage of a small sized goose-quill." The circumference of the opening was dense and white, similar in appearance to the auriculoventricular zone. The septum ventriculorum was deficient at the base; so that a communication existed between the sinus of the right and the cavity of the left ventricle, by which the blood must have passed from the right ventricle into the aorta.

Shortly after Mr. Clark's case was read at the Medico-Chirurgical Society, I communicated a very similar instance of malformation which fell under my notice at the Royal Free Hospital. The following are the particulars of this case.

CASE 5.[1]—*Supernumerary Septum in the right Ventricle; Contraction of the Orifice of the Pulmonary Artery; Aorta arising above an aperture in the Septum Ventriculorum; Death from obstruction of the trunk and branches of the Pulmonary Artery.*

William Holland, a milk-boy, aged fifteen, was admitted under my care into the Royal Free Hospital, on the 20th of February 1847. He stated that on the 13th he had bruised the left knee by a fall, and had since suffered from constant pain in that joint, and also, for two or three days before admission, in the right knee. The day after the accident he began to experience pain in the left side of the chest, and difficulty of breathing.

When admitted, he was much collapsed, and the extremities were cold and livid. The cheeks were of a deep purple colour,

---

[1] Med.-Chir. Trans. vol. 30, 1847, p. 131. The preparation of this case is contained in the Victoria Park Hospital Museum, and is numbered B 5. It is engraved in plate 6, fig. 1.

and the lips blue. The fingers and toes were club-shaped, and the nails incurvated, and very dark coloured. The pulse was 124 in the minute and extremely feeble. The tongue was dry and covered with a whitish fur. The respiration was peculiarly rapid and panting, and he was compelled to lie on the back, partly inclined towards the right side, and with his head low. He complained of pain in the region of the heart, palpitation, and difficulty of breathing. Both knee joints were swollen and tender, and there existed a red and swollen patch over the left trochanter.

The chest yielded a clear sound on percussion, except in the præcordial region, where the resonance was impaired over a larger space than natural. The liver could be felt extending a little below the edges of the ribs. The sternum was arched and prominent, more especially towards its base. The respiration was puerile in character and attended with occasional mucous râles. A loud murmur was heard accompanying the impulse of the heart. It was of a soft or blowing character, and was most intense at the cartilage of the third left rib, near the sternum, or at a point half an inch above the nipple, and between that body and the sternum, and the second sound was there inaudible. From this point it continued to be heard very distinctly, though decreasing in intensity, along the upper part of the sternum, in the subclavian and carotid arteries, and on the left of the spine in the interscapular and dorsal regions. It was also heard less distinctly in a line from between the nipple and sternum, towards the middle of the left clavicle. Below the level of the nipple the murmur became shorter and more feeble, and, at the point of pulsation of the apex, towards the epigastrium, and on the right side of the lower half of the sternum, it was followed by a very clear second sound. The boy was much exhausted, and his intelligence so impaired that it was found impossible to collect any satisfactory information of his state of health previous to the present attack. He stated, however, that he had lost flesh and strength and had been very subject to affection of the chest and of a livid complexion, since he was thrown from a cart twelve months before.

These notes were taken about 4 P.M. on the day of admission, and, notwithstanding the free use of stimulants, externally and internally, he gradually sank, and died at 8 o'clock on the following morning. On inquiry, I ascertained that he had always been of a somewhat livid complexion, but was stout, healthy, and capable of a full amount of exertion, till the occurrence of the accident he referred to. He was then riding at the back of a cart when it toppled up and he was thrown out and fell upon his head. He was admitted into the Royal Free Hospital on the 6th of February, 1846, under the care of my then colleague, Mr. Gay, with symptoms of concussion of the brain. He continued there six days, and the only peculiarity observed in his appearance was some slight lividity of the lips. Since that time he had been gradually getting thinner and weaker; he was constantly chilly, and very subject to take cold. He complained occasionally of palpitation, difficulty of breathing, and pain in the region of the heart; and his hands and face were always very blue, but especially so in cold weather, or when he was suffering from affection of the chest. His appetite was generally defective, and he occasionally vomited his food. His father is of a livid complexion, and has a " pigeon breast."

The *post-mortem examination* took place at 4 P.M. on the 22nd, thirty-two hours after death.

The brain was healthy, though much congested. It weighed 49 oz. 4 drachms avoirdupois.

The surfaces of the pleura on the right side were adherent by a small cellular band. The left lung was entirely free. Both lungs were engorged with blood, sparingly crepitant, and contained several masses in the state of pulmonary apoplexy. The bronchial mucous membrane was somewhat reddened.

The pericardium was healthy. The heart weighed 10 oz. It was broader from side to side than from above downwards. Its total circumference was 8½ French inches, of which the right ventricle constituted 4½. The systemic veins were natural. The right auricle was large, and its walls thick. The foramen ovale was closed, with the exception of a small valvular opening capable of admitting a goose-quill. The Eustachian valve was of moderate size. The right auriculo-ventricular aperture measured thirty-nine lines in circumference, and the valves were natural.

F

The muscular column, to which the cords of the anterior fold were attached, was very large and firm. The aperture opened as usual into the sinus of the right ventricle; but this portion of the cavity was separated from the infundibular part, by a thick muscular septum, defective only at its centre, over a space sufficient to admit the forefinger, and perforated by one or two small pores nearer the apex. The former cavity communicated with the aorta by an orifice thirty lines in circumference, situated at its upper side. Its walls averaged 5½ French lines in thickness, and were unusually firm and solid. In places they had undergone the fibro-cartilaginous degeneration throughout their whole extent, and the serous covering externally was opaque. The second or infundibular portion of the ventricle was of smaller capacity than the sinus, and gave origin as usual to the pulmonary artery. Its walls averaged only two to three lines in thickness. The orifice of the pulmonary artery was very small, and was provided with only two valves, which were extremely thick and opaque. The aperture on the ventricular side admitted a ball measuring fifteen lines in circumference. The valves projected into the cavity of the vessel, leaving deep sacs behind them, and by their free borders occasioned further contraction of the orifice, so that it only gave passage to a ball of thirteen lines in circumference.

The coats of the pulmonary artery were much indurated and thickened, and its canal was entirely obstructed by fibrinous coagula. At the sides of the vessel these coagula were of a dirty white colour, and were laminated and firmly adherent to the valves and lining membrane, but towards the centre of the canal they were softer and less decolorized. The obstruction occupied the whole trunk of the artery, and extended a few lines into each of its branches. The smaller vessels were free from disease. The ductus arteriosus was impervious throughout the largest portion of its extent, but had a conical cavity extending two or three lines from the bifurcation of the pulmonary artery. The pulmonary veins were natural. The left auricle was small, and its lining membrane opaque. The left auriculo-ventricular valves were healthy, and the aperture measured thirty-six lines in circumference. The left ventricle was of small capacity ; its walls felt flaccid, and were $3\frac{1}{2}$ to $4\frac{1}{2}$ lines thick. The opening from the left ventricle into the aorta was of about the same size as that by which the vessel communicated with the right ventricle.

The aorta was healthy and very large from its origin to the sulcus marking the point of connection of the ductus arteriosus ; from that point its calibre greatly diminished. The valves were of the usual number, and entirely free from disease. The bronchial and œsophageal branches were somewhat large. The veins and cardiac cavities were distended with blood.

The abdominal organs displayed no appearance of disease, but were much engorged. The liver weighed 45 oz., the spleen $6\frac{1}{2}$ oz., the left kidney $4\frac{1}{2}$ oz., and the right 3 oz. The latter was somewhat mottled.

Since this case was published I have had the opportunity of examining a specimen which exhibits the form of malformation in a more aggravated degree than any other with which I am acquainted. The preparation was shown to me by Mr. Hutchinson,[1] and was removed by Mr. Keyworth of York, from a cyanotic girl, about twelve years of age, who had been extremely susceptible to cold, and incapable of any active exertion throughout her life. The abnormal septum is constituted, as in the former cases, by interlacing muscular columns, and the aperture is only sufficiently large to allow the passage of a small probe, the contraction being increased by fibrinous deposits on the edges. The infundibular portion of the right ventricle forms a cavity about eight lines in length, between the septum and the orifice of the pulmonary artery. The pulmonary artery is somewhat small, and its valves are apparently only two in number. The sinus of the right ventricle is a small cavity communicating above with the right auricle, and separated from the left ventricle only by muscular bands ; indeed, it seems to constitute a portion of the latter cavity. The left auricle opens naturally into the left ventricle. That cavity is very large, and its walls thick. It gives origin to the aorta, and

[1] Path. Trans., vol. 5, 1854, p. 99.

has also an indirect communication with the right auricle. The aorta is of large size. The foramen ovale is entirely closed, and the ductus arteriosus is pervious some distance from the pulmonary artery, but becomes obliterated before its union with the aorta. The auriculo-ventricular and aortic valves are much thickened.

In all the cases just referred to, the development of the supernumerary septum occurred before the division of the ventricles was completed, or at an early period of fœtal life; but this rule does not apply to other instances in which similar septa have been found. In the following case the abnormal partition constituted the only defect in the development of the heart.

CASE VI.[1]—*Supernumerary Septum in the right Ventricle; Heart otherwise well formed.*

A female child, aged five years, was brought under my notice on the 20th of December, 1846. She was stated to have been livid from birth, but acquired a more natural colour soon after, and was stout and healthy till between two and three years of age; she then began to suffer from difficulty of breathing without any assignable cause, had a slight cough, and became thinner. Since that period she had continued delicate, and was very susceptible to cold. When chilled or suffering from catarrhal symptoms, she became livid in the face, and had hurried and difficult breathing. She was repeatedly seen and examined during the year 1847. At that time her cheeks were tumid and much flushed, the vessels being distinctly visible. The arms and hands were puffy, and the fingers and toes club-shaped at their extremities, and of a deep red or purple colour, but not blue. The pulse was always more or less accelerated. There was some difficulty of breathing, and a slight hacking cough. The dull space at the præcordia was somewhat greater than natural, but the chest was elsewhere fully resonant. Slight sibilant and sonorous râles were heard

---

[1] Med.-Chir. Trans., vol. 31, 1848, p. 61. The preparation of this case is contained in the Victoria Park Hospital Museum, and is numbered B 2. It is engraved in plate 5, fig. 2.

with the respiration, and over a large portion of the front of the chest a loud systolic murmur was audible. This murmur was thought to be most intense midway between the left nipple and sternum; but it was also very distinct from this point towards the middle of the left clavicle, across the sternum to the right side, and along the whole of the middle and lower part of the sternum. In these situations the diastolic murmur was indistinct, but, at the upper part of the sternum, and at the point of pulsation of the apex of the heart, the murmur was less intense and prolonged, and the diastolic sound clear. A feeble murmur was audible to the left of the spine, in the interscapular region. There was no permanent turgidity or pulsation of the jugulars. The liver was large, and the abdomen tumid. In September, 1847, the child returned from the sea-side, where she had been for six weeks or two months, greatly improved in general health. The murmur, however, though less intense, was still audible, and the lividity equally marked. Soon after this she took scarlet fever, had severe ulceration of the throat, followed by vomiting of blood in large quantities, and died exhausted in about three weeks.

The body was examined on the 2nd of November. It was much emaciated. There were slight old adhesions at the lower and posterior part of the left lung, and some lobular condensation in both lungs. The smaller bronchial tubes contained a little secretion, but the mucous membrane was not materially reddened. The heart was of natural form. It weighed $3\frac{3}{4}$ oz. avoirdupois. There was a slight deposit of fat on the surface of the right ventricle, and some old adhesions between the aorta and pulmonary artery. The right auricle was large, and distended with imperfectly coagulated blood. The foramen ovale was completely closed. The right auriculo-ventricular aperture admitted a ball measuring in circumference thirty-nine French lines: the valves were natural. In the cavity of the right ventricle there existed a septum, dividing the sinus from the infundibular portion; and this septum was perforated by an oval aperture, twenty-one lines in circumference, by which the two divisions of the cavity communicated. The edges of the aperture were smooth, and on the auricular side the lining membrane and muscular structure around had undergone the fibro-cartilaginous transformation. The walls of the sinus of the ventricle had an average thickness of two lines; those of the infundibular portion. of only one line. The pulmonary orifice had a circumference of 26½ lines. Its valves were natural, and the ductus arteriosus was occluded. The left cavities were natural ; but the left auriculo-ventricular aperture and the orifice of the aorta, were smaller than the corresponding orifices on the right side. The liver and spleen were large. Both kidneys were extensively diseased, mottled with purple patches, and very lacerable.

A very similar case to that which has just been related has recently been published by M. Claude Bernard,[1] which occurred in a female 56 years of age, who had suffered from an attack of acute rheumatism twenty years before, and died with the usual symptoms of cardiac asthma and dropsy. On examination, the left side of the heart was found healthy, but there was great hypertrophy of the right ventricle ; and, in the infundibular portion of the cavity there was a ring composed of firm, resistant fibrous tissue, which would admit the point of the little finger, and had a diameter of only 10 or 12 millimetres. This septum was situated at least a centimetre below the valves of the pulmonary artery. The orifice and valves of the artery were natural but its trunk was dilated, and the heart presented no other defect except the general enlargement. M. Bernard ascribes the production of the constriction, in this case, to endo-carditis occurring at the time of the rheumatic attack. From, however, the similarity of the defect to that which existed in the former instances, and from the circumstances that in the girl whose case has just been related the symptoms had been noticed from early life, and that in the other instances there were undoubted malformations, it is more probable that the ring was due to irregularity of development. The obstruction may have been only first manifested or materially aggravated after the rheumatic attack. In reference to one of the other cases, it has been suggested that the septum was due to

[1] Arch. Gén. de Méd., 5me serie, t. 8, 1856, p. 167.

hypertrophy of the muscular columns consequent on the contraction at the pulmonic orifice. There was, however, no obstruction at the pulmonic aperture in either of the latter cases, or in those of Mr. Holmstead, Dr. Theophilus Thompson, and Mr Le Gros Clark, in all of which the orifice and valves of the pulmonary artery were healthy. The only explanation applicable to the whole of the cases of this description is that they are examples of irregular development, the deviation from the natural conformation taking place at different periods of fœtal life.

The preparation of Mr. Clark's case is contained in the museum of St. Thomas's Hospital, and is numbered 576. There is also in the museum another preparation, which affords a very good example of this description of malformation combined with defect in the septum. It is numbered 576[a], and is stated to have been removed from a child.

II.—MALFORMATIONS PREVENTING THE HEART UNDERGOING THE CHANGES WHICH SHOULD ENSUE AFTER BIRTH.

PREMATURE CLOSURE OF THE FŒTAL PASSAGES.

In some cases the heart has been found incapable of maintaining extra-uterine life, in consequence of the faulty development caused by the closure of the foramen ovale or ductus arteriosus in the fœtus.

The first recorded instance of *premature closure of the foramen ovale*, is that related by Vieussens, in 1715.[1] The child which was the subject of the malformation lived thirty hours, and when born appeared healthily formed and well nourished, but during its short life had difficulty of breathing, a leaden hue of the surface, and cold extremities. The right ventricle and pulmonary artery were extraordinarily developed, and there was no trace of the foramen ovale. Recently two other cases of this description have been recorded in this country. The first of these occurred in the practice of my friend Mr. E. Pye Smith,[2] in a male child which was well formed and healthy looking at the time of birth, but within five minutes became livid, and had difficulty of breathing. It then lapsed into coma, and died in twenty-one hours. The fossa ovalis was in its natural situation, and was entirely closed by a reticulated membrane, which formed a pouch projecting towards the left auricle. There was a mere vestige of the Eustachian valve. The right auriculo-ventricular aperture, the right ventricle, and the pulmonary artery, were of unusually large size; while the left auricle, and the left auriculo-ventricular and aortic apertures, were very small, and the left ventricle was nearly obliterated. The ductus arteriosus was large, and opened into the aorta somewhat more directly than usual.

[1] Traité de la Structure et des Causes du Mouvement du Cœur, ch. 8, p. 35 quoted by Corvisart, " Essai," troisième édition, 1818, p. 315.
[2] Path. Trans., vol. 1, 1846-47, 1847-48, p. 52.

The other case is reported by Dr. Vernon,[1] and is very similar to that of Mr. Pye Smith so far as the obliteration of the foramen ovale was concerned; but the septum ventriculorum was deficient over a considerable space, so that the aorta arose from both ventricles. The right cavities, as in the former cases, were largely developed; the left, on the contrary, were small. The infant survived four hours and a half. It was very livid during life, and died in convulsions.

The *ductus arteriosus may also become obliterated* at different periods of fœtal life. At least it is by no means unusual in malformed hearts, for no remains of the duct to be found, and this may be referred to that portion of the branchial arch having become abortive at an early period. Thus the duct may be absent when the septum of the ventricles is very imperfect, though two distinct vessels arise from the cavity; and it may also not exist in cases where the development of the organ is more advanced, the septum of the ventricles being only slightly defective. Of the former condition I have already quoted an example recorded by M. Thore;[2] of the latter, cases related by Knox, Blackmore, Lexis, Huss,[3] and Deguise and Aran,[4] afford instances. When the ductus arteriosus is prematurely closed, the pulmonary artery gives passage during fœtal life only to the very small proportion of blood which then circulates through the lungs, and is in consequence so imperfectly developed as to be incapable of conveying the larger quantity which should be transmitted after birth. The small size of the vessel thus becomes a source of permanent obstruction, which entails other defects in the development of the organ. Such seems to have been the origin of the malformation in some of the instances referred to, and the following case affords another example of the same kind.

---

[1] Med.-Chir. Trans., vol. 39, 1856. p. 299.

[2] See page 15.

[3] See references to these cases at pages 49-51.

[4] For references, see page 62.

CASE VII.[1]—*Smallness of the Pulmonary Orifice and Artery; absence of the Ductus Arteriosus ; defect in the Septum of the Ventricles ; Foramen Ovale open.*

The preparation of this case was obligingly forwarded to me by Dr. Bentley, and I am further indebted to him for the following particulars of the patient during life.

When the child was first born, it was noticed to be very livid, a fluttering was perceived at the heart, and the respiration was very imperfect. These symptoms continued for several days, after which it became less livid, but it never acquired the natural colour. About seven weeks after birth, the child began to suffer from attacks of extreme dyspnœa, during which its breathing was rapid and laborious ; it threw its head back and gasped for breath ; its complexion became almost black, and it cried incessantly. These fits subsided after loud stridulous breathing, and the child became cheerful ; but they were brought on by the slightest excitement, and especially on taking the breast or food. At first the fits only occurred about once daily ; but towards the close of life there were sometimes many in the day,—on one occasion fully thirty. The sounds of the heart were not well observed, but there was apparently no murmur ; the beats were, however, rapid and violent, and the radial pulse weak. Till the last month the child was fairly nourished, but it afterwards became extremely emaciated. It died when twelve months and three or four days old.

The child was born at the full period, and of healthy parents. It was their fifth child, and another was said to have something the matter with its heart.

On examination, the membranes and substance of the brain were found congested, and at the base there was some recently effused lymph. There was a large effusion of serum in the ventricles, and some beneath the arachnoid. The lungs were much congested, and in places solid, as if unexpanded.

[1] Path. Trans., vol. 7, 1856, p. 83. The preparation is contained in the Victoria Park Hospital Museum, and is numbered B 9.

The heart weighed $2\frac{1}{2}$ oz. avoirdupois. The right ventricle was larger, and its walls thicker and firmer, than those of the left. The aorta arose from both ventricles, there being a large deficiency in the inter-ventricular septum. The pulmonic orifice was only eight lines ‘in circumference. The valves were two in number, and they were thick and indurated. They were protruded forwards into the artery, so as to form a funnel-shaped aperture from the ventricle, and to leave deep sinuses behind the folds. The pulmonary artery was throughout of very small size, and no traces of the ductus arteriosus could be detected. The foramen ovale was largely open, and the Eustachian vale was very perfect. The ascending aorta was of large size, and suddenly became smaller after giving off the left subclavian artery.

In reference to this case, it might be supposed that the primary deviation from the healthy process of development was the imperfect condition of the pulmonic valves; but this is not probable. Obstruction at the pulmonic orifice, though it may occasion defects in the ventricular and auricular septa, so far from causing the premature obliteration of the duct, would rather occasion the persistence of that passage. It seems, therefore most probable that the primary error consisted in the obliteration of the duct at an early period of fœtal life. The smallness of the pulmonary artery thus occasioned, might entail the defect in the valves, or they may have been involved in the original error.

Closely allied to the forms of malformation which have just been alluded to, are those in which other passages of the heart, which should be permanent, are found wanting. Of obliteration of the pulmonary orifice I have already spoken. The *absence of the right auriculo-ventricular aperture*, has also been incidentally mentioned as noticed in one of the cases described by M. Thore[1], in the case of Mr. Holmes[2], and in a preparation in the museum of St. Thomas's Hospital.[3] In a case of partial transposition of the arteries and veins, related by Dr. Worthington,[4]

---

[1] P. 20.   [2] P. 27.   [3] P . 20.
[4] American Jour. of Med. Sc., vol. 22, 1838, p. 131.

which occurred in a female child twenty-two months old ; and in a case described by Dr. Favell,[1] in which the pulmonary artery was found without valves and the foramen ovale was largely open, in a boy eight years old, the right auricle and ventricle had also no connection. A similar condition existed in the heart of a child which lived nine weeks, exhibited at the Pathological Society, by Dr. Sieveking, in 1853.[2] The septum of the ventricles was defective, the foramen ovale was largely open, and the right ventricle, which gave origin to the pulmonary artery, had no communication with the left auricle.

Of obliteration or absence of the left auriculo-ventricular aperture, the cases of Professor Owen and Mr. Clark,[3] and Dr. Vernon,[4] afford examples. A similar defect existed in a heart exhibited at the Société Anatomique of Paris, by M. Parise,[5] and in a case which occurred at Strasburg, and is reported by M. Valette.[6] In the case of Dr. Blackmore,[7] also, the left auriculo-ventricular aperture is said to have been obliterated, but a fissure existed by which the left auricle and ventricle communicated.

Obliteration of the aortic orifice is reported to have been found by Romberg,[8] in a child which lived four days ; and an example of the same defect was exhibited at the Pathological Society by Mr. Canton,[9] in 1849. By the kindness of that gentleman, I have had the opportunity of examining the specimen. The cavity of the aorta extends nearly up to its origin, but the vessel there becomes entirely impervious, apparently from the adhesion of the valves, so that there is no communication between the artery and the cavity of the left ventricle. The pervious portion of the aorta received its supply of blood from the right ventricle through the ductus arteriosus and pul-

---

[1] Provincial Medical Journal, vol. 3, 1842, p. 440.

[2] Path. Trans., vol. 5, 1853-54, p. 97. This specimen is preserved in the Museum of St. Mary's Hospital.

[3] Supra, p. 13.   [4] Supra, p. 13.

[5] Bullet. de la Soc. Anat., 12me année, 1837, p. 100.

[6] Gaz. Méd. de Paris, 1845, p. 97.

[7] Ed. Med. and Surg. Jour., vol. 33, 1830, p. 268.

[8] Edinburgh Med. and Surg. Jour., vol. 65, 1846, p. 149.

[9] Path. Trans., vol. 2, 1848-49, 1849-50, p. 38.

monary artery. The septum of the ventricles is entire, and while the right ventricle is very large, the cavity of the left ventricle is nearly obliterated. The foramen ovale is freely open and the left auricle is natural. The subject of the defect was a child which lived two days, and was apparently healthy till seized with the convulsions in which it died.

PATENCY OF THE FORAMEN OVALE AND DUCTUS ARTERIOSUS.

Allusion has before been made to the persistence of the fœtal passages when combined with imperfect separation of the ventricular cavities. It is not, however, only when the septum of the ventricles is deficient, that the foramen ovale and ductus arteriosus continue pervious; but in all cases the persistence of these passages is very generally associated with some obstruction at or near the pulmonic orifice.

When the *foramen ovale remains open*, it may be under the following circumstances :—

1*st*. The opening may be unusually large, and the valve entirely wanting.[1]

2*ndly*. The foramen may be larger than usual, or of the natural size; but the folds may be imperfectly developed, so as to be too small to close the opening.[2]

3*rdly*. The opening may be natural, and the valve may have attained the full size; but the membrane may be very defective, being perforated by one or more larger or smaller sized apertures.

4*thly*. The foramen may be of natural size; the valve may be fully developed, so as to be capable not only of covering the orifice, but of reaching some distance above its upper edge; and the membrane may be entire; but the changes which should occur shortly before and after birth may not have taken place. The cornua of the valve may retain their length and be widely apart, and the fold may hang loosely across the orifice,

---

1 This condition is figured in plate 6, fig. 2, from a preparation in the Museum of St. Thomas's Hospital, numbered 579.

2 This defect is shown in plate 6, fig. 3, from a preparation in the Museum of the Victoria Park Hospital, numbered B 10.

so as to offer but little impediment to the continued passage of the blood from the right into the left auricle.[1]

Of these irregularities, the three first are rarely seen, except when the heart presents other serious defects in its conformation. The latter condition, on the contrary, is found in those cases in which, in an organ otherwise well formed, the foramen has been prevented closing by some source of obstruction to the flow of the blood from the right auricle or ventricle.[2]

The closure of the foramen ovale after birth is generally ascribed to the floating up of the fold of the valve above the margin of the opening ; and to its being retained in apposition with the isthmus, by the pressure of the blood which enters the left auricle after the establishment of the pulmonary circulation. On this theory the non-closure of the orifice has been referred to the undue distension of the right auricle, from the existence of some obstruction to the flow of blood from that cavity, causing the valve to be pushed aside from the septum and preventing the adhesion of the membranes. It is, however, very questionable whether these views are correct, and the process by which the opening becomes closed is so purely passive. On examining the heart in young children, at different periods after birth, it will be found that the obliteration of the passage is effected—

1st. By the shortening of the cornua, and the drawing up of the fold of the valve considerably above the edge of the foramen :

2ndly. By the approximation of the cornua, so that the width of the upper edge of the valve is greatly reduced : and

3rdly. By the diminution of the opening itself.

For the production of these changes special provisions exist :— In the hearts of children a few weeks or months old, muscular fibres can readily be traced proceeding from the fasciculi which form the walls of the left auricle, in the course of the cornua of the valve, to be expanded on the curtain. Of these fibres, those

[1] This condition is shown in plate 3, fig. 3, from the specimen described in Case 8, page 83. The preparation is contained in the Museum of the Victoria Park Hospital, and is marked B 3.

[2] See also observations by Mr. Struthers, in the Ed. Jour. of Med. Sc., vol. 15. 1852, 3rd series. vol. 6,) p. 21. Republished in Anatomical and Physiological Observations, part 1, Edinburgh, 1854, p. 63.

from each cornu go to opposite sides, while others, as described by Senac, pass across the fold, following a course more or less parallel to the upper edge of the valve. It is evident that muscular fibres thus placed, must, when they contract, tend, on the one hand, to draw up the curtain so as to cause it to overlap the edges of the opening, and on the other, to approximate the cornua. The opening itself is bounded by the muscular fasciculi which form the inter-auricular septum, and their contraction must reduce the size of the orifice, as also pointed out by Senac. There is therefore every reason to regard the closure of the foramen as an active process, dependant on the contraction of these different sets of muscular fibres; induced, probably, partly by the traction exercised upon them by the expansion of the cavity of the left auricle, from the increased quantity of blood which enters it after birth; and partly by the more stimulating quality of the blood which reaches the cavity or circulates through the cardiac vessels.[1]

If this explanation of the mode of closure of the foramen ovale be correct, the persistence of the opening in some cases of malformation may not be entirely caused by the undue distension of the right auricle, but may partly depend on the quantity of blood entering the left auricle being insufficient to exercise the due amount of traction, or too imperfectly acted upon by the air to produce the requisite excitement. Cases occasionally occur in which the foramen is found closed, though there must always have existed much greater pressure on the right than on the left side, and such cases do not admit of explanation on the ordinarily received theory. The continuance of undue pressure on the right side of the valve for a considerable period after birth, owing to the imperfect establishment of the pulmonary circulation, may, however, prevent the adhesion of the valve to the margin of the opening, and so cause the persistence of the oblique passages which frequently exist between the cavities.

When the foramen ovale is still pervious, the size of the opening

---

[1] See remarks on the mode of closure of the foramen ovale, by the author, published in the Path. Trans., vol. 4, 1852–53, p. 85. The preparations which illustrate these remarks are contained in the Museum of the Hospital for Diseases of the Chest, Victoria Park.

varies in different cases. It may possess a diameter of half an inch to an inch, or it may be of much smaller size, only consisting of a narrow fissure between the upper edge of the valve and the margin of the foramen. When it is largely open, the Eustachian valve often still exists and is fully developed. There is also generally obstruction at the pulmonic orifice, and this is sometimes extreme. I have already mentioned a case which occurred to M. Bertin, in a female fifty-seven years of age, in which the orifice of the pulmonary artery was reduced by disease of the sigmoid valves, to a passage two and a half lines in diameter; and other scarcely less remarkable instances of contraction might be quoted. The alteration in the form of the heart which ensues in consequence of this condition is very marked, and corresponds with that which has been before referred to as resulting from the pulmonic obstruction, when the septum of the ventricles is imperfect.[1] There is, however, some difference in these changes, according to the degree of obstruction and the freedom of communication between the auricles. In some instances, where the contraction at the pulmonic orifice is great and the foramen ovale largely open, the right ventricle is found small and its walls flaccid, and the hypertrophy and dilatation are chiefly manifested on the left side;[2] and this is especially the case when the right auriculo-ventricular aperture also is contracted.[3]

A case of the description of malformation now referred to was related by Morgagni in 1761.[4] It occurred in a girl fifteen years of age, who had been ailing throughout her life, and suffered from shortness of breath and debility, and was generally livid. The heart was small and rounded at the apex ; the right auricle was much enlarged and its walls thickened, and the foramen ovale was so imperfectly closed that the little finger could be passed through the opening. The orifice of the pul-

---

[1] See page 31.

[2] The case of Dr. Hallowell, Am. Jour. of Med. Sc., vol. 22, 1838, p. 366, affords an example in point.

[3] This occurred in the case of M. Bertin.

[4] De Sed. et Causes Morb., Venetiis, 1761, tomus primus, f. 154, and Alexander's translation, 1769, vol. 1, Letter 17, arts. 12 and 13, p. 435.

monary artery was contracted owing to disease of the valves, which were cartilaginous and in places osseous, and were so connected together as to leave only an aperture sufficient to admit a barleycorn. In 1783, Tacconi[1] related an instance of the same defect to the Academy of Sciences of Bologna, which he met with in a girl fifteen years of age, who had been livid, incapable of active exertion, susceptible to cold, and subject to dyspnœa, cough, and expectoration, mixed occasionally with blood. In 1805, a similar malformation was found by Seiler,[2] in a man twenty-nine years of age ; in 1810, by Schuler,[3] in an infant ten weeks old; and in 1817, by Poliniere,[4] in a boy of fifteen. In the latter case the symptoms did not appear till after eight years of age ; the boy then began to manifest the usual signs of malformation, and he had repeated attacks of bronchitis and hæmoptysis, during which he became very livid. The right auriculo-ventricular aperture was also found contracted. Since the last date cases of a similar kind have been reported by Cherrier,[5] Bonnissent, Obet and Pinel ;[6] Bertin and Lallemand,[7] Hallowell,[8] Lombard,[9] Craigie,[10] Spitta,[11] Leared,[12] Struthers,[13]

[1] Comment. Bonon, t. 6, 1783, p. 64.

[2] Horne's Archiv, 1805 ; Hein, obs. 29

[3] Dissert. de Morbo-Cœruleo, Œniponte, 1810 ; Hein, obs. 35.

[4] Bibliothèque Médicale, t. 57, 1817 ; Gintrac, obs. 44.

[5] Thèse, 1820, No. 252, p. 24 ; Gintrac, obs. 48, in a male 34 years of age.

[6] Rev. Méd., t. 6, 1821, p. 175, Gintrac, obs. 50me, in a female 5 years of age.

[7] Recherches sur l'Encephale, 1825, t. 2, p. 7 : Gintrac, obs. 52, in a female 51 years of age, with contraction of the right auriculo-ventricular aperture.

[8] American Journal of Med. Sc., vol. 22, 1838, p. 366, in female child 6 months old.

[9] Mem. de la Soc. de Phys. et d'Hist. Nat. de Geneve, t. 8, 1839, p. 503, in a female 28 years old.

[10] Ed. Med. and Surg. Jour., vol. 60, 1843, p. 271, in a male of 20.

[11] Med.-Chir. Trans., vol. 29, 1846, p. 81, in a female 40 years of age.

[12] Dublin Journal of Medical Science, N.S., vol. 10, 1850, p. 223. The subject was a boy, 8 years of age. The foramen ovale was unclosed over a small space, and the valve itself was defective.

[13] Ed. Monthly Jour. of Med. Sc., 1852, 3rd series, vol. 6, p. 21, and Anatomical and Physiological Observations, part 1, Edinburgh, 1854, p. 63. In a child which lived 15 months. In this case it is stated that the ductus arteriosus was not obliterated but was incapable of transmitting blood.

and Speer;[1] and the following case which occurred in my own practice, was related at the Pathological Society in 1847.[2]

CASE VIII.—*Contraction of the Orifice of the Pulmonary Artery; communication between the Cavities of the Auricles by the Foramen Ovale; Septum of Ventricles entire.*

A young man, twenty years of age, by trade a pipe-maker, was admitted into the Royal Free Hospital under my care, on the 20th of May, 1847. He stated that he had enjoyed good health till two years before. Since that time he had been declining in strength, and had suffered from cough, difficulty of breathing, palpitation and pain in the left side of the chest. He was occasionally observed to be somewhat livid in the face, and had expectorated a considerable quantity of blood six weeks before. He had never had rheumatic fever.

When admitted into the hospital he was delicate-looking, and emaciated; his face pale, and the expression of countenance anxious. The lips were slightly livid, the fingers long and a little clubbed at their extremities, and the nails incurvated and somewhat dark-coloured. He had urgent dyspnœa and a severe cough, and expectorated a large quantity of muco-purulent fluid. The pulse was quick and feeble. The sternum was prominent, and its lower end was directed to the left side, so as to occasion a decided projection of the third, fourth, fifth, and sixth left cartilages, and a corresponding flattening of those of the opposite side. Beneath the right clavicle the chest was contracted and imperfectly resonant, and on the left side it was fuller and more sonorous. The respiratory sounds were masked by subcrepitant and mucous râles. The liver was considerably enlarged. The præcordial dulness commenced above at the level of the third left cartilage, and extended transversely from the right side of the sternum to beyond the line of the left nipple, and there the second sound was

[1] Med. Times and Gaz., N.S., vol. 11, 1855, p. 412. in a female 17 years of age.
[2] Pathological Transactions, vol. 1, 1846–47, 1847–48, p. 200. The specimen is preserved in the Victoria Park Museum, and it is numbered B 3. It is engraved in plate 3, figs. 1, 2, and 3.

entirely masked by it. It was also heard very loudly between the sternum and nipple, and thence towards the middle of the left clavicle. At the top of the sternum it was less distinct and of shorter duration, so that it was followed by a clear second sound. To the right of the lower part of the sternum, there was heard first an imperfect systolic sound, and this was followed by, or lapsed into, a short murmur, which again was succeeded by a clear diastolic sound. A purring tremour was felt in the præcordia. There was no anasarca.

During the time the boy was in the hospital, he continued to sink gradually, and died eleven days after admission.

On examination of the body, the brain was found healthy, but the skull afforded a very marked instance of the unequal growth of the two sides often observed in ricketty children.

The right lung was extensively permeated by tubercle, and towards the apex, contained several small cavities. There was much solid tubercle in the left lung. The bronchial mucous membrane was reddened and the tubes contained much muco-purulent fluid.

There was a considerable amount of serum in the cavity of the pericardium, and the attached membrane was in several places covered by rough and thick patches of old lymph. The heart was situated more towards the left side than usual, and the right ventricle was turned forwards, so that it constituted the whole exposed part of the organ ; while the left ventricle was situated entirely posteriorly.

The heart was of large size, and weighed 12 oz. avoirdupois.[1] The valves of the pulmonary artery were adherent together so as to form a complete diaphragm, extended across the opening into the vessel and perforated in the centre, by an irregular triangular aperture of sufficient size to admit the passage of a lead pencil. This membrane was protruded forwards so as to project into the cavity of the vessel, and displayed three ridges marking the former points of separation of the valves, with deep sacs between each. Around the aperture there was a ring of small vegetations. The right auricle and

---

[1] The weight should not have exceeded 8½ to 9 oz.

ventricle were greatly dilated, and their walls hypertrophied. The parietes of the ventricle measured near the pulmonic orifice, four French lines in width. The muscular substance was unusually firm. The right auriculo-ventricular valves were natural. The foramen ovale was so widely open as to allow of the passage of a ball measuring three French lines in circumference. The Eustachian valve was of large size. The left auricle and ventricle were, relatively to the right cavities, small in capacity, and the walls of the latter were of moderate thickness and flaccid. The aortic and mitral apertures and valves were natural. The ductus arteriosus was impervious. The liver, spleen, and kidneys, were of large size. The glands of Peyer in the ileum displayed small tuberculous depositions, and, in places, commencing ulceration.

In the malformations of which the cases now related and referred to afford examples, the foramen ovale appears to remain open in consequence of the obstruction at the pulmonic orifice. Instances are, however, occasionally met with, in which with an open state of the foramen ovale, the pulmonary artery and orifice are free from disease, and there is no source of obstruction to which the defect can be ascribed. A case of this kind, which has frequently been quoted, was related by Dr. Spry, in 1805.[1] The foramen ovale was so largely open as to be two inches in circumference, and the ductus arteriosus was also pervious. There appears to have been no obstruction in the pulmonary artery or at the outlet of the right ventricle. The subject of the case was a cyanotic female, seventeen years of age. In the museum of St. Thomas's Hospital there is also a preparation illustrating the same condition. It is numbered 579, and is stated to have been removed from a female, twenty-one years of age, who, since she was three months old, had presented characteristic symptoms of malformation of the heart, cyanosis, palpitation, dyspnœa, faintings, occasional convulsive attacks, and lividity. The foramen ovale is so largely open as to have a diameter of fully one inch, and the valve is entirely

---

[1] Memoirs of the Medical Society of London, vol. 6, 1805, p. 137.

wanting ; the heart being otherwise free from disease, except some thickening of the mitral valve. The opening in the inter-auricular septum in this case is figured in plate 6, fig. 2. I have also given a drawing of an imperfectly closed foramen ovale, from a preparation which exists in the collection at the Hospital for Diseases of the Chest, Victoria Park.[1] It was removed from a girl, eight years of age, who was under my care at that institution. She was reported to have been always delicate but to have had no serious disease till she took measles, two years before her death. She died with the usual symptoms of cardiac asthma, and there was no decided cyanosis at any period of her illness. On examination, the valve of the foramen ovale was found very imperfect, so that an aperture remained sufficiently large to admit the passage of the fore-finger. The aortic orifice and aorta were small. The pulmonary orifice and artery were, on the contrary, much larger than usual.

In this case it is doubtful what may have been the cause of the imperfect closure of the foramen. It is possible that the small size of the aortic orifice may have occasioned it ; but it is much more probable that the smallness of the aorta resulted from some obstruction in the pulmonary branches or lungs, which, though showing its effects in the dilated pulmonary artery and open foramen ovale, had itself disappeared. The imperfect closure of the foramen ovale may, indeed, depend on a variety of causes. The most frequent are, doubtless, obstruction at the pulmonic orifice, in the right ventricle, or at the right auriculo-ventricular aperture ; but impediments to the flow of blood through the lungs, or obstruction at the left auriculo-ventricular aperture, or at the orifice of the aorta, would probably equally prevent the obliteration of the passage.

It has been shown that, though the patency of the foramen ovale generally co-exists with some form of obstruction in the right ventricle or pulmonary artery, such is not always the case. It occasionally also occurs that even marked obstruction

---

[1] Victoria Park Museum, B. 16. This specimen is described in the Path. Trans., vol. 2, 1848–49, 1849–50, p. 183.

at the pulmonic orifice is found when the foramen ovale is entirely impervious, and the heart is in every other respect natural. Instances of this kind have been recorded by Philouze,[1] Burnet,[2] Fallot,[3] Craigie and Graham,[4] Tiedemann and Fohman,[5] and Ogle,[6] and a specimen affording a remarkable example of the same condition was exhibited at the Pathological Society in 1852, by Dr. Hamilton Roe. In reference to several of these cases it may, and has indeed, been contended, that the disease of the pulmonic valves was not congenital. From, however, the precise similarity of the changes to those which are found in instances of undoubted malformation, I am disposed to believe that the union of the valves in these cases takes place during intra-uterine life; though there can be little doubt that, when the symptoms do not manifest themselves till late in life, the defect, if congenital, must have been originally slight and have been greatly aggravated by subsequent disease. Such an extreme degree of contraction of the pulmonic orifice as occurred in some of these cases, could certainly not have existed at the period of birth without preventing the occlusion of the foramen ovale.

I have already mentioned that the valve of the foramen ovale does not always become entirely adherent to the edges of the fossa, so that a space is left which admits of the passage of some small or flat body, as a probe or the handle of a scalpel, from the one auricle into the other. Under ordinary circumstances the obliquity of this passage entirely prevents the flow of blood along it; but it has been thought that when the right auricle is greatly distended and the fossa much enlarged, the fold may cease to overlap the upper edge and the passage be

[1] Bulletin de la Soc. Anat., t. 1, 1re année, 1826, p. 158.

[2] Journal Hebd. de Méd., 1831, quoted by Bouilland, Traité, etc., 2me ed., t. 2, p. 281, obs. 28. In a female 7 years of age.

[3] Quoted from a Belgian Journal in Lond. Med. and Surg. Jour., vol. 5, 1834, p. 61, in a female 63 years of age.

[4] Ed. Med. and Surg. Jour., vol. 60, 1843, p. 271, in a man 44 years of age.

[5] Ibid., vol. 65, 1846, p. 127, in a man 21 years of age. Referred to in analysis of Tiedemann on arctation and closure of arteries.

[6] Path. Trans., vol. 5, 1853-54, p. 69, in a female 14 years of age.

restored. Laennec contended that "a blow, fall, or violent exertion might cause the dilatation of the oblique opening;"[1] and a case related by Corvisart[2] has been referred to as an example of an open condition of the foramen ovale so produced. A postilion, fifty years of age, after having received violent blows on the epigastrium, suffered from symptoms of cardiac disease; with great dyspnœa and lividity, and after death the heart was found much enlarged, and an opening existed between the auricles capable of admitting the points of four fingers. I possess a preparation,[3] removed from a female aged fifty-four, who died óf old and extensive disease of the lungs combined with bronchitis, in which the membrane closing the oval opening is expanded into a sac of considerable size, which projects into the left auricle. The valve is not entirely adherent to the margin of the fossa, so that an oblique passage from the right to the left auricle exists. The fold, however, still overlaps the edge of the fossa, and the passage of blood between the two cavities must have been effectually prevented. This specimen therefore shows that the valve itself yields to pressure more readily than it allows of being drawn down; and it is probable that, when a communication occurs in after life between the two auricles, it is rather due to the rupture or erosion of the valve, than to the restoration of the passage. In M. Corvisart's case the opening appears to have been produced by the destruction of a portion of the valve; and M. Bouilland strongly maintains that, in some cases, the communications which take place between the auricles are the result of disease. In a preparation of partial aneurism of the heart which I possess,[4] the valve of the foramen ovale is perforated by a large aperture, probably produced by endocarditis and erosion. There can seldom, I think, be any difficulty in distinguishing cases of this kind from those in which the opening in the septum of the auricles is of congenital origin.

[1] Diseases of the Chest, Forbes' translation, 4th edition, 1834, p. 575.

[2] Essai sur les Maladies du Cœur, 3me ed., 1818., p. 290., obs. 44.

[3] Victoria Park Hospital Museum, C. 20.

[4] Victoria Park Hospital Museum, C 23 ; Ed. Med. and Surg. Jour., vol. 66, 1846, case 1., p. 263.

Patent Ductus Arteriosus.—I have already mentioned that when the orifice or trunk of the pulmonary artery is obliterated, the ductus arteriosus very generally remains open and forms the means by which the blood is conveyed to the lungs. When also there is only some contraction of the pulmonic orifice the passage not unfrequently continues pervious. I shall have shortly to speak of the very general persistence of the arterial duct when the origins of the main arteries are transposed, and the commencement of the descending aorta is contracted or obliterated. At present I propose only to refer to the open state of the ductus arteriosus when that condition is found in hearts otherwise well formed, and where the passage has been prevented closing by the existence of some obstruction at the time of birth.

The closure of the duct is effected by a process of general contraction, which commences at the aortic extremity and gradually advances towards the bifurcation of the pulmonary artery. It is completed at the aortic end while the duct remains pervious at the pulmonic extremity, and thus presents a fusiform cavity, having its apex near the aorta and its base opening into the pulmonary artery. This partially pervious state of the duct is occasionally seen in cases of malformation of the heart where the process of closure has been delayed.

When the duct remains open it may be found of larger size than is usual at the time of birth, as in the cases before mentioned in which the foramen ovale was obliterated during intra-uterine life. It may retain its natural size, as when the aorta beyond the left subclavian artery is greatly obstructed or impervious. It may be reduced to a narrow canal only capable of admitting a probe, a crow-quill, or a small goose-quill. Or lastly it may be found to present a sacculated dilatation, as in a case mentioned by Billard,[1] and of which examples appear to have occurred to Baron,[2] Martin,[3] and Parise.[4]

The length and form of the duct also may vary :—It may

[1 & 2] Maladies des Enfans nouveaux nés, Paris, 1828, p. 567, with a plate.
[3] Bullet. de la Soc. Anat., 2me année, 1827, p. 17.
[4] Ibid., 12me année, 1837, p. 95.

retain its natural length, or be considerably shorter than usual, or may be represented only by a direct opening between the pulmonary artery and the arch of the aorta, as in the case reported by Lediberder.[1] Its position also may be irregular; the most common deviation being, that instead of proceeding from the bifurcation of the pulmonary artery to the descending aorta, below the origin of the left subclavian artery, it arises from the left branch of the pulmonary artery, and is inserted into the aorta opposite the left subclavian artery, or at a still higher point.[2] Indeed it would appear that the under portion of the aortic arch does not become developed in proportion to the growth of the upper part, from which the vessels to the head and upper extremities are given off; and thus in the adult, the cord of the obliterated duct is generally found attached to the under part of the aortic arch, instead of to the descending aorta below the left subclavian artery. In yet other cases the distribution of the duct may be irregular, so that it may give off the left subclavian artery, as in the cases recorded by Holst[3] and Hildenbrand;[4] or, as in one before quoted from Breschet, there may be two ducts, one proceeding from the left pulmonary branch to the aorta, the other from the right pulmonary artery to the brachio-cephalic trunk. In a case observed by Wrisberg,[5] the duct arose as a distinct vessel from the right ventricle.

In cases like those last alluded to, the patency of the duct is combined with the irregular distribution of the vessels from the faulty development of the branchial arches; but more commonly the vessels are regularly developed, and the duct remains open in consequence of some obstruction to the transmission of the blood through the lungs or systemic vessels; and, as these causes would also determine the persistence of the foramen ovale, the patency of the two passages is not unfrequently coincident.

I have already related two cases in which, with an imperfect state of the inter-ventricular septum, the duct remained un-

---

[1] For reference, see p. 60.
[2] See plate 4, fig. 3, and plate 5, fig. 1.   [3] p. 49.
[4] p. 50.   [5] Hein, obs. 67.

closed, and the observations recorded by Obet, Haase, Cheevers, Graves, and Houston, may be referred to as furnishing examples of the same condition. In the cases of Seiler and Schuler, the septum of the ventricles was entire but the foramen and duct were both open. In all these cases the patency of the duct was due to the existence of obstruction to the exit of the blood from the right ventricle at the time of birth. It is probable, also, that contraction of the right auriculo-ventricular aperture, and imperfect expansion of the lungs, by preventing the free circulation of the blood after birth, would equally determine the patency of the duct. In 1846 I exhibited a specimen at the Pathological Society,[1] in which the foramen ovale was partly open and its closure had probably been prevented by the latter cause. A case mentioned by Richerand,[2] in which the septum of the ventricles was imperfect and the duct unclosed, with the pulmonary artery very wide, in a person forty-one years of age, may have depended on the former existence of obstruction in the pulmonic circulation; and the case of Dr. Spry probably affords another example of the same kind. Contraction of the left auriculo-ventricular aperture and of the aortic orifice may also prevent the closure of the duct. A case is related in the Transactions of the Pathological Society of Dublin, by Dr. Mayne,[3] in which the foramen ovale and duct were open, probably from disease of the left auriculo-ventricular aperture, which was so contracted as only to admit two fingers, while the pulmonary orifice admitted three and the right auriculo-ventricular aperture four fingers. The subject of the affection was a female, twenty-seven years of age, who suffered from dyspnœa and palpitation, with a short dry cough, but did not display the slightest cyanosis. The foramen ovale was sufficiently large to allow a half-crown to pass through, and was apparently unprovided with any valve.

In the first volume of the Pathological Transactions,[4] a case

---

[1] Transactions, vol. 1, 1846-47, 1847-48, p. 6.

[2] El. de Physiologie, 1811, t. 1, p. 295.

[3] Transactions, 1847 to 1852, p. 35. Also Published in the Dublin Quarterly Journal of Medical Science, vol. 5, No. 9., N.S., 1848, p. 46.

[4] p. 55.

is related by Dr. Barlow, which occurred in the practice of Dr. Babington, and is possibly an example of an open ductus arteriosus dependant on aortic obstruction. The aortic orifice was of small size, and the valves were four in number. They were extensively diseased and not only caused obstruction to the flow of blood from the ventricle but were incompetent to prevent its return. There was a contraction of the aorta beyond the left subclavian artery, and below this point an opening as large as a goose-quill formed a direct communication between the aorta and pulmonary artery. The patient, a female, thirty-four years of age, was born at the seventh month and suffered from symptoms of cardiac disease from early life. She had never had acute rheumatism.

In some cases, also, the duct and foramen ovale remain open without there being any cause to which the defects can be assigned, and it has been thought that this is more likely to be the case when the child is born before the full period, and is placed in unfavourable hygienic circumstances during early infancy.

III. MALFORMATIONS WHICH DO NOT INTERFERE WITH THE FUNCTIONS OF THE HEART, BUT MAY LAY THE FOUNDATIONS OF DISEASE IN AFTER LIFE.

IRREGULARITIES OF THE VALVES.

Deficiency in the number of the Semilunar Valves.—1*st*. When the number of the semilunar valves is defective, there may be only one curtain, which is stretched across the orifice, or protruded forwards in the course of the vessel so as to assume a funnel shape. When this is the case the fold displays on its upper side three distinct septa or frena (or as they have been termed by John Hunter *cross-bars*[1]), dividing the same number of deeper or shallower sinuses, and indicating the former lines of separation of the several valves by the fusion of which it is formed. The aperture is generally situated in the centre of the fold, and has usually a triangular shape. This condition I have already described as common in the valves of the pulmonary artery and as often co-existing with other serious defects in the development of the heart; but it also, though more rarely, occurs in the aortic valves, and in hearts otherwise well formed.[2]

2*ndly*. In by far the most frequent form of malformation of the semilunar valves, there are two segments, and the deficiency is apparently due to the adhesion of the contiguous sides of two of the original three valves and the atrophy of the corresponding angle of attachment. The former separation of the fused valves is generally indicated by the disproportionate size of the united segment, by the existence of a frenum or band dividing it more or less completely on the upper or aortic side, and usually also

---

[1] Descriptive Catalogue of Pathological Specimens contained in the Museum of the Royal College of Surgeons, vol. 3, 1848, p. 199. Note in reference to No. 1548, quoted from John Hunter's MS. *"Dissections of Morbid Bodies."* This specimen is figured in Baillie's Illustrations of Morbid Anatomy, Fasc. 1, plate 2, fig. 3 ; and similar specimens are engraved in Carswell's Pathological Anatomy, Hypertrophy, plate 2, fig. 4; Hope's Illustration of Morbid Anatomy, fig. 74 ; and Cruveilhier Anatomie Pathologique, 28 liv. pl. 4, fig. 2.

[2] See plate 2, figs. 3 and 4 ; plate 3, fig. 2 ; and plate 4, fig. 1.

by a slight sulcus running across its ventricular surface from
the attached to the free edge and often terminating in a small
notch. The fibrous zone of the united curtain also presents
two more or less distinct crescentic edges.[1] This form of defect
is frequently seen both in the aortic and pulmonic valves.

By most pathologists this condition of the valves has either
been referred to the occurrence of disease in after life ; or to
the breaking down of the angle of attachment from injury
during violent muscular efforts. But while both of these causes
may occasionally produce a blending of two curtains into one, the
defect described is shown to be of congenital origin, at least in
many instances, by its co-existence with other obvious malformations, and by its occurring in children which survive
birth only for a short period and even in fœtuses which have
never breathed. It seems probable that the inequality in the
size of the two existing valves indicates the period at which the
segments forming the united curtain become adherent. When
the two segments are of nearly equal size, the fusion probably
has occurred at an early stage of fœtal existence ; when there
is considerable difference in size, at a more recent period.

3rdly. The third and least frequent form of defect is that
in which there are two large segments, with a small rudimentary
valve interposed between them. This condition probably results
from one of the segments becoming the seat of disease during
fœtal life or early infancy, and so having its further development
arrested.[2]

[1] See plate 1, fig. 3 ; plate 2, fig. 2 ; plate 4, fig. 2, and plate 7, fig. 1.
The last drawing shows a case of fusion of two of the aortic valves, from a
child which died when ten weeks old. There was also a contraction of the
aorta distal to the origin of the left subclavian artery, and the descending
aorta arose in great part from the pulmonary artery. See also fig. 2, plate
7, which shows the union of two of the aortic valves, from a boy aged
fifteen, who was killed. Both these preparations are contained in the
Victoria Park Museum, and are numbered B 17, and B 14. Fig. 3, plate 7,
shows two aortic valves, from a specimen in St. Thomas's Hospital Museum.
This defect in the valves is figured by J. F. Meckel, De cordis conditionibus
abnormibus, Dissertatio Inauguralis, Halæ, 1802, tab. 2, figs. 2 and 3.

[2] See plate 7, fig. 4, from a specimen in St. Thomas's Hospital Museum,
removed from a man 60 years of age, under the care of Dr. Bennett. The
larger valves are extensively diseased. Notes of this case are published in
Pathological Transactions, vol. 3, p. 289.

In most of the cases of deficiency in the number of the semi-lunar valves which I have examined, proofs have been presented of the originally triple form of the apparatus. I do not however deny, that cases occur in which no such evidence of former division can be detected ; but the absence of such signs does not show that they have never existed. For if as we occasionally see, two valves may be of nearly equal size and the indications of the former division of one of them may be only traceable on very careful examination ; or if when a rudimentary valve exists, it may be extremely small and imperfect, we can readily understand that, in some cases, all traces of the original condition of the valves may disappear, though the mechanism of the malformation may have been similar.

The forms of defect now described, though not necessarily interfering with the functions of the heart, do, in a considerable number of cases, lay the foundations of disease in after life.

1st. When the whole of the segments are fused together or when two only are united, the valves not unfrequently become the seat of chronic inflammation, by which they are rendered thick and unyielding and which often goes on to the production of extensive ossification; thus inducing, first obstruction to the flow of blood from the ventricle into the aorta, and then incompetency, by which the blood which has entered the aorta is allowed to regurgitate into the ventricle. This process is often so slow in its progress, that the ventricle accommodates itself to the additional exertion required; and the disease becomes a source of manifest evil only after the lapse of many years, when the valves have become so immoveable as not to allow of the transmission of a sufficient column of blood into the aorta, or so much reduced in size as not to be capable of preventing its return ; when the ventricle is no longer capable of performing the extra labour required to overcome the obstruction ; or when the effects of more acute disease are superadded to the original valvular defect.

2ndly. When two of the valves are united, the line of fusion, or of former separation, is less readily extensible than the other parts of the united fold ; and thus that portion does not expand with the progress of growth so as to accommodate itself to the natural enlargement of the orifice, but is as it were held back, and leaves an open space between its edge and the other segment, by which the blood regurgitates from the aorta[1] into the ventricle.

3rdly. The tendency to regurgitation in the latter class of cases, and also in the instances in which the fold does expand equally in all parts, is increased by the want of the support to the edge of the larger curtain which should be afforded by the corresponding angle of attachment. The edge of the valve thus becomes retroverted, and regurgitation from the aorta into the ventricle is either aggravated or occasioned. In the Edinburgh Monthly Journal of Medical Science, for 1853,[2] I have reported several cases of disease of the aortic valves which originated in one or other of these ways.

Excess in the number of Segments of the Semilunar Valves.— Specimens displaying redundancy of the semilunar valves less frequently occur than those in which the number of the curtains is defective ; and while the latter condition is probably most common at the aortic orifice, it is the valves of the pulmonary artery which are most frequently in excess. Of forty-one cases of irregularity of the semilunar valves which I examined and reported upon at the Pathological Society in 1851, nine only exhibited excess in the number of segments, and in eight of them the irregularity existed at the pulmonic orifice.

The chief forms in which this description of irregularity existed in the specimens which I have examined, have been :—

1st. Four segments ; three of nearly equal size, and a smaller one interposed between two others and generally imperfectly separated from one of those to which it is adjacent.[3]

2nd. Four segments of nearly equal size, or with two larger

---

1 This defect in the valves is referred to by Dr. Brinton, as existing in a specimen exhibited at the Pathological Society in 1855: Path. Trans., vol. 5, p. 72.

2 On Malformation of the Aortic Valves as a cause of Disease.

3 Plate 8, fig. 1, from a preparation marked B 13, in the Museum at the Victoria Park Hospital. The valves are the pulmonic, and the subject of the peculiarity was a female 75 years of age.

than the other two, and in either case with two of the segments imperfectly separated.

3rd. Four segments; one distinct, and three more or less blended together.[1]

4thly. Three or four segments of nearly equal size, with one or two smaller curtains interposed between others, and imperfectly separated from those to which they are adjacent.[2]

Where the number of the semilunar valves is in excess, the redundancy would appear to be due to the more or less perfect subdivision of one or more of the segments. Thus, in some cases, the curtains of the valves are blended together; and in others the angle of attachment of one of the segments is wanting, and the septum interposed between the two sacs is defective, being either perforated by larger or smaller apertures, or almost entirely wanting.

In the absence of any exact information as to the process of development of the semilunar valves, it is not easy to offer a satisfactory explanation of the cause upon which the excess in the number of segments depends. The peculiar arrangement of the apparatus in some fishes may however afford an indication of the mode in which the valves are formed in man. In the preparation of the heart of *Cephalopterus Giorna* (Cuv.), or American Devil Fish, contained in the museum of the Royal College of Surgeons,[3] three muscular columns are seen to extend the whole length of the bulbus arteriosus, from its commencement in the ventricle to its termination in the branchial artery. At a short distance from the ventricle small valvular folds

[1] Plate 8, fig. 2. Drawing of the pulmonic valvular apparatus in a specimen which I have not retained. It was removed from a man aged 45, who was crushed to death.

[2] This condition is illustrated in plate 8, figs. 3, 4, and 5. Figure 3 shows four aortic valves from a specimen in the Museum of St. Thomas's Hospital; fig. 4, shows the defective state of the septum between two of the valves, at the point marked *a*. It is doubtful whether the small body marked *b* is a rudimentary valve, or merely a band of false membrane. Fig. 5, is a good example of five pulmonary valves, from a preparation marked B 12, in the Victoria Park Museum. The specimen was removed from a female 4½ years old. Excess in the number of the pulmonic semilunar valves is figured by Meckel in tab. 2, fig. 1.

[3] No. 910 of the Physiological Series.

H

project from the sides of each muscular column, so as to form six imperfect valves, and of these there are several rows. The folds become more distinctly valvular as they advance towards the branchial artery, till at the termination of the bulbus arteriosus, they appear as three well formed semilunar valves. Each muscular column terminates at the base of one of these valves, so that it would seem as if the latter were formed by the approximation and blending of two of the folds, the muscular column becoming at the same time abortive. A very similar arrangement of the valves in the bulbus arteriosus obtains in other cartilaginous fishes, as the Grey Shark, *Galeus Communis*, (Cuv.), and the Skate, *Raia Batis*, (Linn.). It is probable that the semilunar valves in man may be developed in a mode analogous to this; each curtain consisting originally of two portions, which are ultimately blended together, and lose their central attachment to the sides of the orifice. This suggestion is in accordance with the fact that when more than the proper number of segments exist, the excess is apparently due either to one or more supernumerary curtains being attached to other segments, or to the imperfect division of some of the curtains. If this supposition be correct, the increased number of valves, so far from depending on excessive development, results from arrest of growth :—the condition being thus analogous to other forms of malformation which apparently depend on excessive development, though they really indicate the arrest of the process at a rudimentary stage, as has been before shown to be the case when a supernumerary septum exists in the right ventricle. It does not appear that excess in the number of the semilunar valves materially interferes with the efficient performance of their functions. It is possible that the curtains may less readily apply themselves to the sides of the aorta and pulmonary artery during the ventricular systole, when there are four or five segments, than when the usual number exists. If so the condition may be the cause of some obstruction to the flow of blood from the ventricle into the artery. The results of subsequent disease are however certainly much less frequently seen in such cases than when the number of the segments is defective.

The semilunar valves are also occasionally found to present a condition to which the term *atrophy* has been applied ; the segments, chiefly at the free edges, and especially towards the angles of attachment, presenting small apertures, or spaces in which the fibrous tissue is wanting and the continuity of the curtain is only maintained by the two folds of endocardium. Sometimes, also, strong fibrous bands are found extending from the angles of attachment to different parts of the free edges of the curtains. This condition is common in valves which are otherwise irregular, especially when the number of the segments is in excess, and will be found figured in the plates.[1] In these cases, therefore, it is doubtless a congenital defect; but it is probable that in some instances it may occur in after life from the stretching and distension of the valve. It probably does not ordinarily interfere with the action of the valves, and is therefore an unimportant change.

MALFORMATIONS OF THE TRICUSPID AND MITRAL VALVES.

The three segments of the tricuspid valve are occasionally found united together, so as to form a kind of membranous septum stretched across the right auriculo-ventricular aperture, and perforated in the centre by a larger or smaller opening, generally of a triangular form. This condition closely resembles the first description of malformation of the semilunar valves ; and though usually considered as resulting from disease in after life, is, I suspect, really of congenital origin. It occasionally exists in combination with other decided malformations, as in instances reported by Lallemand and Louis,[2] and one which I have related in this work ;[3] and when this is not the case there are often other circumstances which indicate its con-genital origin. Two cases of this kind have fallen under my notice. In one of these, related by Mr. E. Pye Smith, in the Pathological Transactions,[4] the patient had been ailing all her

---

[1] Plate 8, fig. 1 *a*, fig. 5 *b, c*, and especially fig. 4 *c*.

[2] Memoires ou Recherches Anatomico-Pathologiques. Communication des Cavités Droites et Gauches, obs. 6 and 10. See also references at pp. 50 and 82.

[3] p. 47.

[4] Vol. 3, 1850-51, 51-52., p. 283.

life, and, though thirty-seven years of age, did not appear to be more than fifteen or sixteen, and had never presented any signs of puberty. She was feeble both in body and mind. She had never had rheumatism, or other affection likely to have been complicated with disease of the heart. In the other case, the patient, who was under my own care at the Aldersgate Street Dispensary, was thirty-two years of age, and had suffered from two attacks of rheumatic fever, the first thirteen, the second two years before she fell under my notice. Since the former seizure her symptoms had been aggravated; but she was distinctly stated to have laboured under palpitation and dyspnœa prior to the first attack, and indeed from her earliest infancy. In both these instances the mitral valves were also adherent, and the orifice greatly contracted; and in a case recorded by Mr. Burns, and one referred to by Laennec,[1] and regarded by him as possibly resulting from intra-uterine disease, a similar complication existed. If therefore it be correct to regard the fusion of the curtains of the tricuspid valve as of congenital origin, it becomes probable that some of the cases of union of the folds of the mitral valve, also depend on changes taking place during fœtal life. The only author who, so far as I am aware, has previously expressed this opinion, is Mr. Burns,[2] and his remarks on the subject have attracted little attention. From, however, the complete fusion of the folds of the mitral valve which is sometimes found; from the occasional co-existence of this condition with the similar disease of the tricuspid valve and with decided malformations of other parts of the heart; and from the early age of the persons in whom this disease occurs in its most characteristic form, I cannot but believe that Mr. Burns's views are, at least in some cases, correct. This inference is corroborated by the facts that the auriculo-ventricular apertures are occasionally obliterated during fœtal life, and that both the tricuspid and mitral valves have been found to present evidences of recent inflammation in newly born

[1] Diseases of the Chest, Forbes's translation, 4th edition, 1834, p. 574.

[2] Diseases of the Heart, 1809, p. 28, quoted by Farre, On Malformations, p. 42.

children, and even in the fœtus.[1] It is true that generally
in cases of great contraction of the auriculo-ventricular
apertures, the patients have at some periods of their lives
laboured under rheumatism, and that their symptoms have
either originated or become seriously augmented subsequent to
such attacks. This is, however, as has been several times remarked, often the case in instances of undoubted malformation,
and is in accordance with the general pathological law, that
whenever a part has once been the seat of disease it is ever
after prone to take on similar action, during which any injuries
which it may have sustained in the first attack become
greatly aggravated. I, however, throw out these remarks rather
as suggestions to be confirmed or disproved by future observations, than as established views.

The mitral and tricuspid valves also occasionally present a
condition similar to that which in the semi-lunar valves has
been termed "*atrophy.*" The curtains are found unusually short,
and display portions in which the fibrous tissue is wanting, or
the valve is perforated from the giving way of the two layers of
endocardium. This cribiform condition is chiefly seen towards
the free edges of the valves, and especially of the attached
curtain of the mitral. It is probably sometimes a congenital
defect, and in other cases occurs in after life from the yielding of
the folds when unduly stretched. It may, in some cases, be a
cause of incompetency.

Among the malformations which may predispose to disease
in after life, may be classed the cases in which the walls and
cavity of the left ventricle are disproportionate to the size of
the aorta—a condition which has been supposed by Corvisart,
Laennec,[2] and some others, to be a congenital defect. There
is, however, reason to doubt the correctness of this view;
the disproportion referred to being probably the result of
irregular growth after birth.[3]

---

[1] See case by Dr. Massmann of Berlin, quoted in Arch. Gén. de Méd., 5me
serie, t. 5, 1855, p. 80, in which the mitral and tricuspid valves presented
recent disease in an infant which lived only twenty hours. The sounds of the
fœtal heart before birth had been replaced by a loud bruit.

[2] Treatise on Diseases of the Chest, trans. by Forbes, 4th ed., 1834, p. 534.

[3] See Observations on Certain Diseases Originating in Early Growth, by Dr.
Barlow, in Guy's Hospital Reports, vol. 6, 1841, p. 235, and vol 7, 1842, p. 467.

The heart has in some cases been found too small. This condition has been supposed to be congenital, and Otto[1] informs us that he has met with very small hearts in cases in which there were other malformations, as well as in infants and grown-up persons in whom the organ was otherwise well formed, and he refers to similar observations recorded by Kerkring, Morgagni, Kreyzig, &c.

The external form of the heart has also been found in some cases irregular, without the organ being otherwise defective. Thus Bartholinus[2] reports that he has found the apex bifid, and the heart of an infant displaying the same condition was exhibited by M. Parise at the Société Anatomique of Paris in 1837.[3]

[1] Pathological Anatomy, South's translation, p. 264, sects. 1 and 2.

[2] Paget on Congenital Malformations. Ed. Med. and Surg. Jour., vol. 36, 1831, p. 281.

[3] Bulletin, 1837, p. 100.

IV.—MALFORMATIONS CONSISTING IN THE IRREGULAR DEVELOPMENT OF THE PRIMARY VESSELS.

TRANSPOSITION OF THE AORTA AND PULMONARY ARTERY.

In this malformation the points of origin of the primary vessels are transposed, the pulmonary artery arising posteriorly from the left, and the aorta anteriorly from the right ventricle. The first case of this kind with which I am acquainted is that described by Dr. Baillie in the second edition of the Morbid Anatomy, published in 1797,[1] and figured in the engravings, and of which the preparation is in the possession of the Royal College of Physicians. It occurred in the practice of Dr. Wollaston, of St. Edmundsbury. The child died when two months old, and was remarkably livid and cold during life, but did not suffer from dyspnœa. The arteries were transposed, the ductus arteriosus was sufficiently large to admit a crow-quill, and the foramen ovale was a little more closed than in a new-born infant. The heart was of a natural size for a child of the age, and was otherwise healthy. In 1811 Mr. Langstaff[2] related a similar case, in which the infant, immediately after birth, was of a dark purple colour in the face, and of a brownish black in other parts of the body. When three weeks old he began to suffer from attacks of dyspnœa, and died suddenly in one, seven weeks after. The condition of the heart was very similar to that in the case of Dr. Baillie. In 1814, Dr. Farre[3] recorded a case in which the child lived five months; and since that time others have been reported by Wistar,[4] Gamage,[5]

[1] P. 38. Works by Wardrop, vol. 2, p. 36. Engravings, plate 6, fasiculus 1st.

[2] London Medical Review, vol. 4, 1811, p. 88, quoted in Farre, on Malformations, p. 28.

[3] On Malformations, p. 29.

[4] System of Anatomy, 1814, Philadelphia, vol. 2, p. 78, in a child 2½ years old.

[5] New England Journal of Med. and Surg., 1815, Boston, vol. 4, p. 244, in a child 15 weeks old.

Tiedemann,[1] Duges,[2] Coliny,[3] King,[4] Walshe,[5] &c.; and in 1851, a specimen of this kind of malformation was exhibited at the Pathological Society, by Dr. Ogier Ward,[6] which I had the opportunity of examining. It was removed from a child which was livid from the time of birth, had a feeble cry, took the breast with difficulty, was sleepy, and had irregular respiration. It died on the 18th day. The aorta arose from the right ventricle, and the pulmonary from the left; the septum of the ventricles was entire, and the duct and foramen were both pervious. The child died of congestion of the brain, and the lungs were found engorged and imperfectly expanded.

Transposition of the vessels may occur in combination with the corresponding misplacement of the heart and other viscera, as in the instance related by Mr. Gamage, or when the heart occupies its natural position, as in by far the larger number of cases. It may be found in hearts which are otherwise imperfectly formed, the septa of the ventricles or auricles being largely defective, as in the case of M. Thore,[7] and in a preparation which is contained in the Museum of St. Thomas's Hospital;[8] when the septum of the ventricles is only defective to a slight extent, as in the cases of Coliny, Stedman, and King; or

[1] Zeitschift für Physiologie, Heidelberg, 1824. 1 band, p. 111, with plate. The infant lived 12 days.

[2] Journal Gén. de Méd., t. 101, 1827, p. 88, in a child 4 or 5 days old.

[3] Arch. Gén. de Méd., 2me serie, t. 5., 1834, p. 284. In a male infant, which lived 2 years and 7 months.

[4] Med. Gaz., 1841, child lived 2 years and 9 months.

[5] Med.-Chir. Trans., vol. 25, 1842, (N. S. vol. 7), p. 1, in a male infant, which lived 10 months.

See also Martin, Müller's Arch. für Anat. und Phys., 1839, p. 222, with plate; in a child which lived 10 weeks.

Johnson, American Journal of Med. Sc., vol. 46. (N. S. vol. 20), 1850, p. 370; in a male infant which lived 2 months.

Ducrest, Arch. Gén. de Méd., 3me et nouvelle serie, t. 9, 1840, p. 76; in a female, which lived 10 hours.

Stedman, Lancet, 1841–42, vol. 1, p. 645, with sketches; in a female child, which lived 7 months and 8 days.

Stoltz, Gaz. Méd. de Paris, 22 année, 1852, 3me serie, p. 154, quoted from Gaz. Méd. de Strasbourg, 2 cases; 1st case, an infant which lived 5 days; 2nd case, an infant which lived 37 days.

[6] Path. Trans., vol. 3, 1851–52, 1852–53, p. 63.

[7] Referred to at p. 20.   [8] Referred to at p. 20.

when the septum of the ventricles is entire. The last is the most common condition, and occurred in ten out of thirteen cases of which I have collected notes, and it is stated by Dr. Chevers to exist in a preparation contained in the Museum of Guy's Hospital. In most instances the arteries only are misplaced; but in some, as those of Farre, Gamage, Walshe, and Stoltz, the ventricles, as indicated by their relative size and by the form of the auriculo-ventricular valves, are also transposed. In a case not included in the previous enumeration, reported by M. Boyer,[1] in which the viscera generally were reversed, the venæ cavæ entered the left auricle, and the pulmonary veins the right. The aorta arose above an aperture in the septum cordis, so that it communicated with both ventricles; the pulmonary artery was connected with the right ventricle. The foramen ovale was open, but the ductus arteriosus was not pervious through its entire course. The infant which was the subject of the malformation lived two months. A very similar case, before referred to, is related by Dr. Worthington in the American Journal of Medical Sciences.[2]

In some cases of transposition the arteries and veins are also irregularly distributed: thus, in one related by the late Mr. T. W. King there were only two pulmonary veins; in that of Dr. Walshe there were two carotid and two subclavian arteries, and in that of Mr. Gamage the aorta followed an unusual course, making its turn to the right, and passing down on the right side of the spine, and forming the arteria innominata on the left side. The venæ cavæ were also situated on the left side. In all the cases of this description of malformation on record, the foramen ovale has been open to a greater or less extent, but in some the ductus arteriosus has been found impervious. This occurred in three out of four instances in which the septum of the ventricles was imperfect, and even when the ventricular cavities are completely separated, the duct has in some cases been found of very small size, and in two it was entirely obliterated. In reference to one of these cases,—that related by Mr. Gamage,—Dr. Chevers suggests that there probably

---

[1] Arch. Gén. de Méd., 4me serie, t. 23, 1850, p. 90, and Gaz. Méd. de Paris, t. 5, 1850, p. 292. This specimen was exhibited at the Acad. de Médecine.

[2] Vol. 22, 1838, p. 131.

existed some communication between the pulmonary veins and the systemic auricle, or some other channel through which the vessels communicated; but in the case of Mr. Wistar it is expressly stated that there was no communication between the aorta and pulmonary artery by the ductus arteriosus, and that the veins entered the auricles as usual. In both cases the foramen ovale was largely open. The child, in the former case, lived fifteen weeks; in the latter, two years and a half.

In 1854, I exhibited at the Pathological Society, a heart, obligingly sent to me by Mr. Wordsworth,[1] which had been removed from an infant under the care of Dr. Hess; and which displayed transposition of the aorta and pulmonary artery in conjunction with other defects. The following report of the case during life was furnished by Dr. Hess:—

"The child was a strong well-developed boy, but had a cough with hurried breathing and palpitation from birth. He had repeated paroxysms of dyspnœa, some of which continued for three hours, and during the attacks he was slightly livid in the face, but not more so than is common in severe bronchitis. He gradually grew weaker and thinner, notwithstanding that the digestive functions were unimpaired; looked old in the face, and at last was a complete skeleton. The extent of the dulness on percussion in the region of the heart was much increased. The heart's sounds were clear, and there was no murmur. The boy died suddenly, when eight months old, in coma preceded by convulsions, which came on after one of the asthmatic paroxyms."

On examination the heart had a quadrangular form. The auricles were completely separated the foramen ovale being entirely closed by its valve. Both auricles opened into the left ventricle—the right auricle on the right, the left auricle on the left side of the cavity. The right auriculo-ventricular aperture was of large size, the left was much smaller. The left ventricle was very large, and, at its upper and posterior part gave origin to the pulmonary artery. The right ventricle was a small rudimentary cavity from which the aorta arose, and which communicated with the left ventricle by a crescentic opening ten lines in circumference. The valves, at the orifice of the pulmonary artery

1 Path. Trans., vol. 6, 1854-55, p. 117.

were of very unequal size ; the ductus arteriosus was not retained
in the preparation, but, from the size of the pulmonary artery,
the passage had probably been pervious.

DESCENDING AORTA GIVEN OFF FROM THE PULMONARY ARTERY.

I have already alluded to the faulty development of the
ductus arteriosus : the pulmonary artery and aorta may also
present irregularities in their distribution. Thus the pulmonary
artery may be divided at a lower point than usual, as in a case
observed by M. Cassan,[1] where the trunk of the vessel was only
three lines in length, and that of Mr. Bloxham,[2] in which it did
not exceed one line. The aorta may be double, as in a case
seen by M. Bertin ;[3] but the most frequent and important irregularity is that in which the aorta, after having given off the
vessels to the head and upper extremities, becomes greatly
contracted or obliterated, or is entirely wanting; so that the
inferior parts of the body derive their supply of blood through
the ductus arteriosus and pulmonary artery.

This form of irregularity, in which the descending aorta is
said to be given off from the pulmonary artery, was first noticed
as existing in two preparations described by Dr. Farre, and
contained in Sir Astley Cooper's museum. The preparations
are now preserved in the Museum of St. Thomas's Hospital,
and have been before referred to as examples of deficiency in
the septum interposed between the left ventricle and the
infundibular portion of the right ventricle, immediately below
the origin of the pulmonary artery. They have on this account
been described by Dr. Farre as instances of the pulmonary
artery deriving its origin from both ventricles.[4]

The child from which one of these preparations was removed,—
that numbered in the museum 1435—is stated to have presented
nothing unusual till a fortnight after birth, when it began to
breathe quickly, and to waste ; the heart pulsated strongly ; the

[1] Arch Gén. de Méd., t. 13, 1827, p. 82.

[2] Med. Gaz., vol. 15, 1835, p. 435. In a female child which lived three
years, in whom the pulmonary artery was very small, the aorta arose from
both ventricles, and the foramen ovale was imperfectly closed.

[3] Maladies du Cœur, 1824, p. 443. The aorta arose singly, but then
divided and reunited to form the descending aorta.

[4] On Malformations, p. 15, 13.

skin was always pale, and the hands and feet cold ; the lower extremities, and occasionally the face, became œdematous, and the
child died suddenly at the age of eight months. The ascending
aorta divided into the arteria innominata, the left carotid, and the
left subclavian arteries, and terminated in a very small trunk,
which was continued into the descending aorta. The pulmonary
artery was larger than the aorta, and arose from both ventricles
(or, more properly, arose from the right ventricle, but communicated with the left through the aperture in the septum),
and, through the medium of the ductus arteriosus, gave off the
descending aorta. The foramen ovale was much dilated. In
the other case, the preparation of which is numbered 1436,
the child during life had hurried and panting respiration,
was of a dark purple colour, and died convulsed when nine
days old. As in the other case, the aorta gave off the usual
branches at the arch, and then formed a small trunk, which
proceeded towards the descending aorta ; but its cavity became
impervious before it united with that vessel. The pulmonary
artery arose from the right ventricle, above an aperture in the
septum ventriculorum, and the ductus arteriosus was continued
into the descending aorta. The valve of the foramen ovale was
very imperfect, and the cells of the lungs were not fully inflated.
In 1847 I exhibited and described at the Pathological Society,
a preparation displaying this irregularity, which was forwarded
to me by the late Dr. G. A. Rees,[1] with the information that it
was removed from an infant ten weeks old, which was thought to
have been born at the eighth month. The child was feeble, and
had much difficulty of breathing from birth. It was never
observed to be livid in the face or extremities, and was indeed
unusually pale. Large portions of the lungs were in the condition of atelektasis. The ascending portion of the aorta was
unusually large, but after giving off the branches at the arch,
the vessel diminished greatly in size, so that between the
origin of the left subclavian artery and the point of communication with the ductus arteriosus, it had scarcely half its former
calibre. After the entrance of the duct, the aorta again ex-

---

[1] Path. Trans, vol. 1, 1846-47, 1847-48, p. 203. The specimen is preserved
in the Victoria Park Hospital Museum, and is numbered B. 17.   It is drawn
in plate 7, fig. 1.

panded, and it retained its acquired size throughout the thoracic portion. The orifice and trunk of the pulmonary artery were large, and the duct was freely open and led directly into the descending aorta. The foramen ovale was closed, and the different valves healthy. The aortic was much smaller than the pulmonic orifice. An instance of malformation very similar to this is described in the same volume of the Transactions by Dr. Chevers,[1] and another was reported by Mr. Barrett[2] in the *Lancet* of 1835. In several instances the ascending and descending aortæ have been found entirely disunited. Thus, in a child which survived birth only for a short time, Steidele[3] found two vasa arteriosa to arise from the heart, one of which—the pulmonary artery—furnished two branches to the lungs, and was then continued into the descending aorta ; while the other—the aorta—formed the carotid and axillary arteries. In 1834, M. Gibert[4] exhibited, at the Société Anatomique, at Paris, the heart of a child which was born at the full period and lived twelve days, being during that time pale and cold, and suffering from dyspnœa. As in the former case, the aorta gave off the vessels to the upper parts of the body, and the descending aorta was derived from the pulmonary artery. The foramen ovale was largely open, and the septum of the ventricles imperfect. A precisely similar condition was also found in a fœtus of the ninth month, described by Mr. Struthers and Dr. Greig.[5]

Of the deviations from the natural arrangement of the large venous trunks, the most frequent are the existence of two ascending or two descending cavæ ; of two, instead of four pulmonary veins, or the irregular insertion of these vessels. Thus the pulmonary veins may enter the right, and the systemic veins the left auricle. The two sets of veins may communicate with the same cavity, or the auricle may be deficient, and the veins may enter the ventricle directly ; but these irregularities are not of sufficient importance to require further notice.

[1] Path. Trans., vol. 1, p. 55.   [2] Lancet 1834 and 1835, vol. 1, p. 349.

[3] Hein, obs. 66.   The other particulars of this case are not reported.

[4] Bullet. de la Soc. Anat., année 14, 1839, p. 203.   Noticed also in Proceedings of Society, an. 7, 1832, p. 108.

[5] Monthly Journal of Med. Sc., vol. 15, 1852 (N. S. vol. 6), p. 29, with woodcut.   See also Anatomical and Physiological Observations, by John Struthers, part 1, Ed. 1854, p. 75.

1. MODE OF FORMATION.

THE malformations of the heart of the first class, are all more or less closely allied, and depend on the process of development being arrested at different periods of fœtal life; so that the organ retains one or other of the forms which are proper to it at different periods of growth.

In some cases, and especially when the heart consists of only two cavities, as in the instance described by Mr. Wilson, we cannot detect any cause to which the arrest of development can be ascribed; but in others, in which the growth of the organ has proceeded to a more advanced stage, we are frequently able to trace the circumstances which have prevented its further development. This will, however, be more apparent, if we reverse the course adopted in describing the various kinds of malformation, and trace the condition of the heart from the more perfect to the more rudimentary forms.

If, during fœtal life, after the septum of the ventricles has been completely formed, the pulmonic orifice should become the seat of disease, rendering it incapable of transmitting the increased current of blood required to circulate through the lungs after birth, the foramen ovale may, as was clearly shown by Morgagni,[1] be prevented closing; and if, as was further pointed out by Dr. Hunter,[2] the obstruction take place at an earlier period, when the septum cordis is incomplete, a communication may be maintained between the two ventricles. The same cause may also determine the permanent patency of the ductus arteriosus; for if during fœtal life the pulmonary artery be much contracted or wholly obliterated, the blood must be transmitted to the lungs through the aorta; and, unless the

---

[1] Letter 17, arts. 12 and 13.
[2] Med. Obs. and Enq., vol. 6. p. 305.

ductus arteriosus be itself obstructed, that vessel will necessarily become the channel by which it is conveyed. Similar effects would result from obstruction in the course of the pulmonary artery, or in the lungs ; in the right ventricle, or at the right auriculo-ventricular aperture. On the contrary, obstruction at the left side of the heart, as at the left auriculo-ventricular aperture, or at the orifice or upper part of the aorta, would cause the current of blood to flow from the left auricle or ventricle into the right cavities, and thence, through the pulmonary artery and ductus arteriosus, into the aorta, so as to determine the persistence of the foramen and duct, or of an opening in the ventricular septum. The pulmonary artery and aorta would indeed appear to be either capable of maintaining for a time both the pulmonic and systemic circulations, and the necessary effect of the one vessel having the twofold function to perform, would be to give rise to hypertrophy and dilatation of the cavities of the heart more directly connected with it, and to the atrophy and contraction of those which are thrown out of the course of the circulation.

These effects must vary according to the period of fœtal life at which the obstruction takes place. If, as has been before shown, the pulmonary artery be obstructed before the complete division of the ventricles, the septum may be made to deviate to the left side, so that the aorta may become connected with the right ventricle, and both the systemic and pulmonic circulation may be chiefly maintained by that cavity. If, on the other hand, the obstruction take place after the completion of the septum, the double circulation will be carried on by the left ventricle :—in the former case the left, in the latter the right, ventricle becoming atrophied. The *degree* of obstruction may also influence the course of the circulation, and so affect the development of the heart. A slight impediment at or near the pulmonic orifice, while the growth of the septum cordis is in progress, will probably give rise to hypertrophy and dilatation of the right ventricle, and to the persistence of a small inter-ventricular communication. More aggravated obstruction, on the contrary, may arrest the process of development and throw the maintenance of the circulation on the left ventricle.

The influence of obstruction, at or near the pulmonic orifice or in some other portion of the heart, in modifying or arresting the development of the organ, is thus far capable of demonstration; but it is probable that similar causes may equally give rise to the more extreme degrees of malformation, in which one or other cavity retains its primitive undivided condition. For if obstruction taking place during the growth of the septum be capable of preventing its complete development, it may be inferred that impediments occurring at a still earlier period, may entirely arrest the formation of the septa, so as to cause the ventricle or auricle or both, to remain single or to present only very rudimentary partitions. It cannot, however, be disputed that, in some cases, more particularly when the arrest of development is extreme, no source of obstruction exists to which the defect can be assigned ; but it must be borne in mind that the absence of any obvious impediment to the circulation after the lapse of a considerable period, as in persons dying several years after birth, does not afford any proof that some obstruction might not have existed when the deviation from the natural conformation first commenced. Indeed, as remarked by Dr. Chevers, the condition which, at first sight, appears least in accordance with the theory of obstruction—that in which the pulmonary orifice and artery are dilated—really affords evidence that some serious impediment must have existed in the lungs or elsewhere, though it may have entirely disappeared.

These inferences seem, indeed, so natural that I should not have thought it necessary to dwell upon them, especially as they have received the support of some of the ablest writers on the subject,—Louis, Williams, Craigie, King, and especially Dr. Chevers,—had it not been that different views have been advanced by M. Bouilland, and more recently by M. Forget. The former author not only contends that the apertures in the septa are frequently due to disease in after life, but ascribes the thickening and induration of the valves which most generally cause the obstruction at the pulmonic orifice, to inflammation occurring after birth and induced by the entrance of aerated blood into the right ventricle. To these views there are insuperable objections. In a large proportion of cases, the pulmonary orifice or artery is so con-

I

tracted as only to allow a small amount of blood to be subjected
to the influence of the air, and thus the circulating fluid must
be chiefly venous, and can have little effect, even if it enter the
right cavities. Very generally, also, the right ventricle is
more powerful than the left, and the blood must flow from the
right to the left side, instead of in the opposite direction as
supposed by M. Bouilland. The cause, therefore, which he
regarded as producing the valvular disease cannot, under ordinary circumstances, operate. There is also conclusive proof,
in some cases, that the valvular disease is congenital; for it has
been found in infants which have died very shortly after birth,
and even in fœtuses which have never breathed ;[1] and in other
instances its intra-uterine origin may be fairly inferred from
the precise similarity of the diseased changes to those which
are clearly congenital.

While, however, I differ in opinion with M. Bouilland, as to
the relation which exists between the pulmonic disease and the
defects in the ventricular and auricular septa, and as to the
period at which the changes at the pulmonic orifice occur, I
fully concur with him in regarding them as due to inflammation. Analogy would lead us to expect what clinical experience
demonstrates,—that the fœtus in utero is liable to diseases precisely similar in their nature and results, to those which affect
the child after birth, and there can be no doubt that both the
peri- and endo-cardium are not unfrequently the seat of inflammation during fœtal life.[2]

This view, however, is not without its difficulties. In after

[1] I have myself found the valves adherent in a monstrous fœtus, still-born,
and in an infant, a girl ten weeks old, in which the disease was evidently of
old date. Specimens have also been obligingly forwarded to me by Mr.
Obré, and Dr. R. Quain showing the disease in infants which died at the ages of
six weeks and six months, and in which there was no appearance of any
recent affection of the heart, and the children died suddenly without having
been previously indisposed. Path. Trans. vol. 4, pp. 96 and 101.

[2] A case by Dr. Massmann of Berlin, in which there was disease of the
mitral and tricuspid valves during fœtal life, has already been referred to.
Billard also relates that in an infant two days old he found strong adhesions
between the laminæ of the pericardium, evidently of old date, and regarded
them as the result of pericarditis during fœtal life.

life valvular disease is most usually situated on the left side of the heart, and when the valves on the right side are also affected, it is to a much less degree. Whereas, in cases of malformation, it is on the right side that the disease is situated. I am indeed doubtful whether the difference which exists is really so great as it appears; but there can be no doubt that during fœtal life, disease is more common on the right than on the left side. If, then, the process of disease at the two periods, be identical, to what is the difference in its seat to be assigned? It cannot depend on the blood which circulates through the right ventricle and pulmonary artery being more stimulating than that which enters the left ventricle and aorta. So far as there is any difference in this respect, as a large portion of the blood which is conveyed to the right ventricle by the ductus venosus and inferior cava, is transmitted through the foramen ovale to the left auricle and ventricle, did this cause operate in the production of disease, its effects would be manifested on the left side. Neither is the function of the right ventricle during fœtal life more active than that of the left; for the blood which enters the right auricle is equally distributed between the two ventricles. Perhaps, however, the more immediate connection of the right ventricle with the circulation in the descending aorta and umbilical arteries, may explain the greater liability to disease at the orifice of the pulmonary artery; for the circulation in the cord and placenta would appear to be more liable to temporary obstruction than that in the body of the fœtus itself. We know that in after life the variable pressure of the blood in the arterial system is a fruitful cause of disease in the aortic valves.

The second form of malformation—that in which the vessels are misplaced or unusually distributed, must be ascribed to the improper division of the bulbus arteriosus, and to the irregular development of the branchial arches.

The transposition of the aorta and pulmonary artery cannot be referred to any deviation from the natural position of the septum cordis. It is not simply that the pulmonary artery arises from the left ventricle and the aorta from the right, but the positions of the two vessels are reversed, so that the pulmonary artery originates from the posterior and upper part of the left ventricle, and the aorta from the anterior and upper part of the right ;—the lower portion of the latter vessel crossing the origin of the pulmonary artery in the same way that the pulmonary artery ordinarily embraces the origin of the aorta. The production of this form of malformation is to be ascribed, as is well explained by Dr. R. Quain, to the irregular division of the bulbus arteriosus, so that the branchial arches ordinarily associated with the portion of the bulb which forms the pulmonary artery, become connected with the aorta ; while the arches which should be associated with the portion of the bulb which becomes the aorta, are in connection with the pulmonary artery. This deviation from the natural development may take place either after the septum of the ventricles is completed or while the growth of the septum is in progress, so that the transposition may involve the ventricles as well as the vessels. The contraction or obliteration of the aorta beyond the left subclavian artery, which occasions the open state of the ductus arteriosus, must be ascribed to the obliteration of that portion of the branchial arch ; and the existence of two arterial ducts, or of two aortæ, is due to the persistence of portions of the arches which should become abortive. Irregularities in the number or position of the large venous trunks admit of explanation in the same way.

In the descriptive portion of this work I have made no allusion to excessive development of the heart; for various malformations which have been regarded as examples of that condition, such as those in which supernumerary septa exist, or where there are two aortæ, or a ductus arteriosus on each side, or two descending or ascending cavæ, really result from defective development; while others are met with only in monstrous fœtuses incapable of extra-uterine life, and are therefore of no practical importance, and as such would be beside my purpose.

The various facts which have been recorded, show that in the heart, deviations from the natural process of development may occur during all stages of fœtal life,—before the division of the cavities has commenced, after it has to some extent progressed, and when it is entirely completed. It is not, however, clear at what period the irregular development most commonly begins. If inferences were to be drawn from the published cases of malformation, this would appear to take place most frequently during the later periods of fœtal life. The correctness of such a conclusion may, however, be doubted. The earlier the period at which the process of development is deranged, the greater will probably be the defect, and the less readily will the system accommodate itself to the change after birth. So that the cases in which, with any marked deviation from the natural conformation, life is maintained for a longer or shorter period, probably constitute only a small proportion of those in which the development is irregular. It seems reasonable to suppose that during the earlier periods of fœtal life, when growth is most rapid, the process would be most liable to derangement.

In the production of defective development, sex has been supposed to exercise an influence, and malformations are certainly most common in males, though why it should be so seems incapable of explanation. I find, however, that of ninety-one cases of malformation which I have collected, and in which the sex of the subjects is recorded, fifty-two were males, and thirty-nine females, or 57·2 and 42·8 per cent. respectively.

The occurrence of accidents and strong impressions upon the mind of the mother, are also supposed to conduce to the irregular development of the offspring, and in many cases such causes appear to have operated. In several instances which have fallen under my notice, the mothers of children labouring under malformations of the heart, have assigned the defect in the children to strong mental impressions or shocks which they sustained during pregnancy ; and there seems reason to believe that such causes, by deranging the fœtal circulation, might produce the effects. In other instances, also, there has apparently been an hereditary predisposition to defective development of the heart, more than one child of the same parents having been affected.

SYMPTOMS.

The symptoms by which malformations of the heart are characterised, are referable to derangement of the circulatory and respiratory functions, and to the secondary disorders of the various viscera so induced. A child, labouring under serious malformation of the heart, generally presents at birth a very livid colour. The respiration is imperfect and difficult, and the heart is observed to beat violently. There may, however, be no unnatural appearance whatsoever at the period of birth, and the symptoms may only present themselves at the expiration of some months, or even years. When once the signs of obstructed circulation have been manifested, they may either be permanent, or they may soon subside and the child may acquire a healthy appearance, and thrive naturally. In either case, however, paroxysms generally occur, in which the breathing becomes extremely difficult, rapid, or gasping; the surface of the body, more especially of the face and extremities, acquires a dark, in some cases, almost a black hue; and the infant indicates by its cries great distress. Not unfrequently it becomes convulsed, and when exhausted by its struggles, the symptoms subside, and disappear more or less completely. The paroxysms recur at longer or shorter intervals, and with varying degrees of severity, according to the extent to which the deviation from the natural conformation of the heart predisposes to embarrassment of the circulation. I find, by a careful analysis of 101 cases of malformation, characterised by well-marked symptoms during life, and in which the period at which the symptoms were first observed is reported, that in 74 cases they were first noticed either at the period of birth or very shortly after; while, of the remaining 27, in 15 they appeared before the expiration of the first year; in 1 at the sixteenth month; in 3 at two years; in 2 at three years; in 1 at three and a half years; in 2 at five years; in 1 at eight years; in 1 at thirteen years; and in 1 at fourteen years of age; and the period which elapsed might be still further extended. In cases, however, in which the symptoms are stated to have been long deferred, it may be doubted whether, during earlier life, there were really no indications of any irregularity about the heart. It is more probable that the period at which the signs are said to have been first manifested, was rather that in which they became so much aggravated as to attract attention. In two cases the symptoms supervened or became much more marked, after falls at five and fourteen years of age.

In some cases, in the intervals between the paroxysms, the action of the heart may not be materially deranged, the pulse being natural, or only displaying some want of power. In others it may be constantly rapid and jerking; and in the paroxysms it frequently becomes intermittent, very irregular in force or frequency, or barely perceptible. The vessels in the neck may beat visibly, and there may be a marked venous pulsation. The impulse of the heart is usually powerful, and an unnatural murmur is generally heard. The condition of the respiration is liable to similar variations. In some cases there may be but little dyspnœa; in others the respiration is at all times rapid and laborious, and it is usually rendered much more difficult by any exertion or excitement. The lividity of the surface may be only slight, so that the lips may be a little purple and the nails discoloured; or even these symptoms may not be present, the child retaining either its natural appearance or being unusually pallid. In other cases, the surface generally is extremely livid and the lips, hands, and feet of a deep purple colour; and the congestion of the capillary circulation is shown by the slowness with which the colour returns into the integuments, after they have been blanched by compression. The peculiar tint of the surface varies from a simply rose or livid colour, to deep purple, blue, or black; the latter being most generally observed in the lips and beneath the nails. The capillary vessels in the cheeks are distinctly marked, and not unfrequently those of the conjunctivæ convey dark blood. The duration of the paroxysms varies from a few minutes to several hours, and they may recur very frequently, or only every two or three days, or still more rarely. Sometimes the attacks are only brought on by active exertion, as when the child is washed or dressed, or on exposure to cold; but, in other cases, the slightest exertion, even that of taking the breast, or any trivial transition of temperature, will be followed by increased difficulty of breathing, palpitation, and lividity. The nurse frequently finds out by experience some mode by which she can relieve the paroxysms when they occur, as by patting the back of the child, or laying it across the lap with its face downwards, so as to compress the chest. The disposition of the infant is generally very irritable; and, if it be thwarted, the paroxysms are immediately brought on. Though occasionally the integuments become infiltrated, so as to give the child a gross appearance, more frequently it is much emaciated. The abdomen is generally tumid and the head large. In a case, however, which has been for some time under my care, in which I have reason to believe there is some serious deviation from the natural conformation of the heart, the head is remarkably small.

If the child survive the period of infancy the symptoms continue similar in character. From the defective respiration the power of generating heat is very feeble, the extremities are cold, and there is peculiar susceptibility to changes of temperature, so that the child is liable, on the slightest exposure, to suffer from bronchitic attacks. The paroxysms of dyspnœa terminating in syncope, are brought on by any unusual excitement of mind, by active exertion, by cold, or by any disorder of the stomach from indigestible food. The children often learn to avoid these causes, so that they do not engage in play with others and prefer a warm fire-side. In some instances they can arrest the progress of the attacks by lying down, or by compressing the chest in any other way against a resistant body. Generally their mental power is very feeble, and not unfrequently they suffer from pains in the head and occasional convulsive attacks, and they are liable to hæmorrhages, and to unhealthy sores in different parts of the body, more particularly on the fingers and toes, and around the anus. Most usually they are thin, and the fingers and toes have a bulbous shape and the nails are incurvated. In some cases of malformation the emaciation is extreme. Dr. Hunter[1] remarks, in reference to the boy whose case he has related, that " though he was remarkably thin, he had not the look of being emaciated by

1 Med. Obs. and Enq., vol. 6, 1784, p. 300.

consumption; on the contrary, it appears to be his natural habit. If a man had never seen any of the canine species but the bull-dog, for example, he would be struck at the first sight of the delicate Italian greyhound. This young gentleman put me in mind of that animal, and when I looked upon his legs particularly, I could not but think of the legs of a wading water-fowl." In females, if they survive to the period of puberty, the catamenial function is rarely established.

Cyanosis.—There are few subjects in the range of medical science which have occasioned more discussion, than the inquiry as to the immediate cause of the discoloration of the surface, which forms so marked a feature in most instances of mal-formation of the heart.

Morgagni, in describing the case to which I have before referred, ascribed the marked cyanosis which had been observed during life, to general congestion of the venous system, caused by the obstruction at the origin of the pulmonary artery, and this view was also adopted by Dr. Pulteney. Dr. Hunter, on the contrary, seeing that in the case which he has related the septum cordis was imperfect, so that the aorta was supplied from both ventricles, and that a large proportion of the blood circulating in the body must have been venous, supposed that the livid colour the boy had presented during life, was owing to the intermixture of the currents of blood. These views have each since met with numerous supporters. The theory which ascribes the production of cyanosis to congestion of the venous system has been advocated by Louis, Ferrus, and Valleix in France; by Hasse and Rokitansky in Germany; by Joy in this country, and very ably by Stillé in America. On the other hand, the view which refers the discoloration to the intermixture of the venous with the arterial blood, has been supported by Gintrac and, with some modification, by Bouilland and Forget, in France; by Meckel in Germany; by Lombard; and by Farre, Paget, Williams, Hope, Crampton, and Walshe, in this country. Corvisart and Laennec appear disposed to adopt the former explanation; and Dr. Chevers, while regarding the cyanosis as chiefly due to congestion, contends for the influence of the venous blood in the arteries, as increasing the intensity of the discolorization.

Gintrac, after a careful analysis of fifty-three cases, in all of which there was more or less intermixture of the currents of blood, inferred that cyanosis is dependent on the presence of venous blood in the general circulation, though he admitted that the intermixture was not always productive of cyanosis. Louis and Ferrus have dwelt more fully on the absence of any constant connection between the intermixture of the currents and the existence and intensity of cyanosis. Dr. Stillé,[1] after a careful examination of a very extended series of cases of different forms of malformation of the heart, has shown, 1*st*, that cyanosis may exist without the intermixture of the currents of blood; 2*ndly*, that there is no just proportion between the intensity of the cyanosis and the amount of venous blood which enters the systemic vessels; 3*rdly*, that complete intermixture may take place without cyanosis being produced ; and 4*thly*, that the variations in the extent, depth, and duration of the discoloration, are inexplicable by the doctrine of the intermixture of the currents. Of 77 cases which he has collected and carefully analysed, he finds the condition of the pulmonary artery reported in 62 ; and that in 53 of these it was contracted, obstructed, or impervious ; while in the remaining 9 cases, there were other conditions present which would give rise to congestion of the venous system. He was therefore led to adopt the view of Morgagni and Louis, and to infer that cyanosis is dependant either on obstruction at the pulmonic orifice, or on some other cause giving rise to venous congestion. This theory he regards as not only satisfactorily accounting for the discoloration of the skin and the dyspnœa and other symptoms, but he contends, that congestion of the venous system is always present when cyanosis exists, and is never found without the occurrence of cyanosis, unless there are satisfactory reasons for its absence.

M. Valleix,[2] one of the most recent writers on this subject,

---

[1] On Cyanosis, or Morbus Cæruleus, by Morton Stillé, M.D., Am. Jour. of Medical Sciences, N.S., vol. 8, 1844, p. 25.

[2] Guide du Médecin Praticien, 3me ed., 1853, t. 1er, p. 738 and p. 27 of this work.

concludes "that cyanosis cannot be regarded as the pathognomonic symptom of communications between the right and left
cavities of the heart, and does not constitute a particular disease;
but is common to several affections and is only more or less
frequent in each of them." He refers to a case under his care
at the Hospice des Enfants Trouvés, in which an infant presented nothing unusual in its appearance, and went through
the ordinary changes after birth, though the septum of the
ventricles was a mere rudiment, and the freest intermixture
of the currents of blood must have existed.

All modern writers either adopt the exclusive views of M.
Louis and Dr. Stillé—that cyanosis depends on venous stasis; or
regard it as partly due to congestion of the venous system, and
partly to the intermixture of the venous with the arterial blood.
Those, however, who uphold the latter theory, differ widely in
the extent to which they suppose the one or the other cause
to operate. Dr. Walshe[1] says, "How is that doctrine (that
cyanosis depends on congestion of the venous system) recon-
cilable with the fact that the most intense obstruction may
occur in the adult without inducing true cyanotic discoloration?
How comes it, too, if communication between the two sides of
the heart be so unimportant, that in five only, out of seventy-
one cases of cyanosis collected by Stillé, was such communication
wanting? Is it not likely that two things, so constantly found
together, act as cause and effect, and that when a widely open
foramen ovale has been found (as it certainly occasionally has)
without previous cyanosis, some corrective condition, either
organic or dynamic, has existed to prevent the intermixture.
Doubtless constriction of the orifice of the pulmonary artery
will increase the darkness of tint, by inducing venous stagna-
tion; but I do not think there is evidence to show that,
unassisted, such constriction can produce cyanosis." Dr.
Speer,[2] who, in a recent number of the Medical Times and
Gazette, has discussed this question, concurs in the views of
Dr. Walshe.

---

[1] On Diseases of Lungs, Heart, and Aorta, 2nd. ed., 1854, p. 713.
[2] 1855, p. 412.

In the previous portion of this work I have alluded to various cases which bear out the inferences of Dr. Stillé. I have mentioned the case of a girl in whom an abnormal septum was found in the right ventricle, without any other malformation of the heart, and who was cyanotic during the several months she was under my observation, affording striking proof that cyanosis may exist without intermixture of the currents of blood. In the case of Dr. Hale, in which there existed only one ventricle ; and in that of Dr. G. A. Rees, in which the pulmonary artery gave off the descending aorta, not the slightest lividity was observed ; so that these cases evince that the freest intermixture may exist without giving rise to cyanosis. Instances exhibiting the occurrence of cyanosis without intermixture, or the free entry of venous blood into the arterial system without cyanosis, are however, much less frequent, than cases which display a want of just relation between the intensity of the lividity and the amount of intermixture. In one of the instances of abnormal septum which I have mentioned as having fallen under my own notice, the aorta arose in great part from the right ventricle, so that a very large proportion of the blood circulating through the body must have been venous ; yet there was no evidence that the boy had presented any material degree of cyanosis till shortly before his death. He had been an inmate of the Royal Free Hospital, for an accident about twelve months before, and nothing unusual was then observed in his appearance. The occurrence of cyanosis was apparently manifested after the pulmonary artery became the subject of disease, by which its capacity was still further diminished. In the case of Dr. Hess also, in which the arteries were transposed, as the auricles both opened into the left ventricle and the right ventricle had no connection with the corresponding auricle, but derived its blood from the left ventricle, the blood circulating in the systemic vessels must always have been, to a great extent, venous ; yet the child was only livid during the paroxysms of asthma, and then not more than is seen in severe bronchitis. The absence of lividity in this case, on the supposition that cyanosis is dependant on congestion of the venous system, is readily explained by the absence of any marked obstruction to the circulation at any of the orifices, so that general venous congestion could not ordinarily have existed. But, on the theory that cyanosis is caused by the mixture of the currents of blood, its absence in the case is quite inexplicable.

The fact that cyanosis is not always observed where abnormal communications exist between the two sides of the heart, has been admitted by the supporters of the theory of intermixture, and various reasons have been assigned for its absence; and especially it has been contended, that, provided the pressure on the two sides be equal, no intermixture will take place, though either septum be defective. To this it may, however, be answered, that the cyanotic symptoms are by no means always congenital, and do not, indeed, sometimes appear till after many years, even when the freest intermixture of the currents of blood must have existed from birth. In cases of this kind, the accession of the cyanosis may generally be traced to the occurrence of disease either in the heart or lungs, by which the original source of obstruction is aggravated. Thus, during a slight attack of rheumatism, inflammation may affect valves previously malformed, so as to curtail still further the size of the opening into the pulmonary artery; or the aperture may be so rigid and unyielding, as not to expand sufficiently with the progress of growth; or an attack of bronchitis, by adding obstruction in the lungs to that which already existed in the heart, may cause the aggravation of cyanosis if previously present, or create it where not before observed.

Lastly, cases frequently occur in which the variation in the degree of lividity cannot depend on any corresponding variation in the amount of intermixture. I recently saw an infant which suffered at intervals from the usual symptoms of malformation of the heart.[1] While quite quiet, there was no appearance of cyanosis, but paroxysms of dyspnœa with great lividity, were readily brought on by exposure to cold, or by excitement or exertion. Under a mild alterative treatment, the paroxysms become less frequent, and had, indeed, ceased entirely, till the child, then three months old, took hooping

[1] See case 3, p. 47.

cough attended with bronchitis, when they recurred with much greater severity, and the cyanosis became intense. On examination after death, the folds of the tricuspid valve were found somewhat adherent together, much thickened and indurated, and studded with recent fibrinous deposits; the right ventricle was hypertrophied and dilated and the pulmonary artery of large size. At the base of the septum of the ventricles there existed two apertures, leading from the left ventricle immediately below the origin of the aorta, into the sinus of the right ventricle. These apertures were larger on the left than on the right side, so that it was evident that the current of blood which had passed through them must have flowed from the left ventricle into the right; and, from their small size, they could neither have given passage to a large current, nor, from their hard and unyielding edges, could the quantity transmitted have been liable to material variation. The cyanosis could not, therefore, have been owing to the venous blood entering the left ventricle, and so being circulated through the body. Neither could the variations in its intensity have been due to any corresponding variation in the amount of intermixture. The different degrees of congestion of the venous system consequent on the increased difficulty in the transmission of blood through the lungs, could alone explain the recurrence of the paroxysms. In this case, also, the left arm and hand were at all times very livid and somewhat swollen; and it was found on examination, that the venous trunks on that side, had been compressed by enlarged glands at the root of the lung and in their course.

From these considerations, we are, I think, warranted in inferring that the cyanosis is due to congestion of the venous system. I cannot, however, concur in the opinion of Laennec, that the lividity in cases of malformation, differs in no degree from that which attends ordinary disease of the heart or lungs: and that in some forms of affection of the lungs, the discoloration of the skin is as considerable and as general as in cases of malformation. The cyanosis of malformation, when very marked, is much more intense than that from any other cause;

but, occasionally, the lividity which attends pulmonary and cardiac disease is quite as intense as in some instances of malformation. In support of this, I may mention the case of a boy, seventeen years of age, who was a patient of mine at the Royal Free Hospital in 1847, and had presented marked cyanosis from early life, yet in whom the discoloration was dependent on imperfect expansion of the lungs, connected with curvature of the spine, and the right ventricle was very greatly hypertrophied and dilated. That in cases of pulmonary and ordinary cardiac disease, the cyanosis is generally so much less intense than where the heart is malformed, is probably to be ascribed to the amount of congestion being also less. In cases of acquired disease, were so small a proportion of blood submitted to the influence of the air, and were the general congestion so extreme, as in many instances of malformation, life could not be maintained. In acute affections, also, the integuments generally become more or less œdematous, so that the lividity is masked.

Dr. Stillé's observations point too exclusively to contraction of the pulmonary orifice as giving rise to the congestion on which the cyanosis is dependent. In the previous lectures, cases have been adduced in which the obstruction was caused by an abnormal septum in the right ventricle. An instance has just been mentioned in which it was dependent on disease of the tricuspid valves; and, as before stated, it is sometimes caused by imperfect expansion of the lungs.

On the other hand, Dr. Chevers has shown, by reference to a case under the care of Dr. Lloyd, that great contraction of the orifice of the pulmonary artery, when it occurs in adult life, is not necessarily productive of cyanosis; and the case of Dr. Hamilton Roe before mentioned, shows that cyanosis is not always caused by even great *congenital* contraction of the pulmonary orifice. A case described by Dr. Craigie and one related in this work, also evince that the cyanosis when present, does not always bear a strict relation to the amount of obstruction. In all exceptional cases of this kind, however, I believe it will be found that the right ventricle has acquired such an increase of power, as to be able to overcome the difficulty in transmitting the blood through the contracted orifice and so prevent the occurrence of general congestion. In my own case, in which the patient died of phthisis, it is probable that the lividity had become less with the gradual diminution in the amount of blood circulating in the body with the progress of the pulmonary disease.

The inferences to be drawn from the facts brought forward appear to be, that while obstruction to the flow of blood through the lungs or from or into the right ventricle, giving rise to general venous congestion, is the essential cause of cyanosis, the intensity of the lividity and its peculiar colour, are modified by other circumstances.

1st, It is probably necessary to the production of intense cyanosis, that, as suggested by Dr. Chevers, the obstruction to the circulation should either have been present before birth, when the capillary vessels are naturally more capacious than in the adult; or, that it should have existed before the full development of the body was attained, and while the entire vascular system was more readily dilatable ; or, at least, that it should have been of long duration, so that the capillary vessels may have become greatly expanded.

2ndly, The condition of the integuments also probably materially affects the production of cyanosis. In cases in which the peculiar blue or black colour is observed, the skin is usually very thin, and the body generally emaciated. Where, on the contrary, the discoloration is rather of a deep rose tint, the patients are not much emaciated, or are even, in some cases, tolerably well nourished ; and, where the skin is pallid, there is either no material congestion, or it is masked by the oedematous condition of the integuments.

3rdly, and lastly. There can be no doubt that the intensity and peculiar tint of the cyanosis must be much affected by the colour of the blood in the vessels. Where a very small portion of the blood can be submitted to the influence of the air in the lungs, the whole mass must be of an unusually deep colour, and the hue of the surface generally will be proportionately dark.

DURATION OF LIFE IN PERSONS LABOURING UNDER DIFFERENT FORMS OF MALFORMATION.

After the description which has been given of the various malformations, it will readily be understood that there is considerable difference in the influence they exert upon the duration of life.

Where there is only some slight irregularity in the development of the heart, so that small openings exist in the septa of the auricles or ventricles, the defect is of very little importance; indeed, it is by no means uncommon for such openings to be found in the hearts of persons who have died at advanced periods of life, and have never presented any signs of cardiac disease. On the other hand, where the arrest in the development of the heart is more extensive, and is combined with some form of obstruction, it becomes a source of serious suffering and the duration of life is necessarily limited to a comparatively short period.

In those cases in which there is *moderate contraction of the orifice or trunk of the pulmonary artery, while the heart is otherwise well formed,* the increased power of the right ventricle may so far overcome the difficulty in transmitting the blood through the lungs, as to maintain the balance of the circulation, and allow a considerable amount of health and vigour to be enjoyed for many years. This was well illustrated by the case related at the Pathological Society, by Dr. Hamilton Roe, in which the patient lived to the age of thirty, and had been noted for his performances as a pedestrian. The patient under the care of Dr. Graham in the Edinburgh Infirmary, survived to the age of forty-four, and had been able to follow his employment of a navigator, working on one of the railways, till six weeks before his death. In another case reported by M. Fallot, the patient attained to sixty-three years of age. In this description of cases, however, the congenital origin of the disease is open to doubt.

Where *the foramen ovale is open,* the obstruction at the pulmonary orifice is generally greater than in the class of cases just mentioned, and the duration of life is therefore less. In-

K

stances, however, have occurred in which the patients have survived for many years. Of 15 persons presenting this form of malformation of whose cases I possess notes, 10 are recorded to have lived to the age of fifteen years and upwards. Of these, 6 died at the ages of twenty, twenty-eight, twenty-nine, thirty-four, forty, and fifty-seven; and my own patient survived to the age of twenty. In 3 cases the ductus arteriosus was open, and the subjects of the malformation attained the ages of ten months, fifteen months, and twenty-nine years.

Where, with *contraction of the pulmonary orifice, the septum cordis is imperfect,* so that the aorta has a more or less direct communication with the right ventricle, and the obstruction must have occurred at an early period of fœtal existence, the duration of life is still further curtailed. Of 52 such cases, 12 only survived the age of fifteen; and of these, 2 died at the age of sixteen, 1 at seventeen, 1 at eighteen, 1 at twenty, 2 at twenty-one, 1 at twenty-two, 1 at twenty-three, and the remaining 3 at twenty-five years of age. In the four cases related in the previous portion of this essay, death took place at seventeen months, two years and five months, six and a-half years, and nineteen years. In cases of this description, the open state of the foramen ovale and the imperfection in the ventricular septum, so far from adding to the danger, really afford the means of relief to the overcharged right auricle and ventricle, without which life could not be prolonged for any considerable period. It does not, however appear, that, provided the septum of the ventricles is imperfect, the closure of the foramen ovale materially affects the prospects of longevity. The mean duration of life in the cases in which the septum of the ventricles was imperfect and the foramen ovale open, and in those in which apertures existed in the septum cordis and the foramen was closed, having been nearly equal. In only eight of the fifty-two cases was the ductus arteriosus pervious, and in these, one of the patients died at the age of seventeen months, 1 at two years, 2 at three years, 1 at seven years, 1 at nine years and eleven months, 1 at thirteen years and a-half and one at nineteen years.

Where the *pulmonary artery is entirely impervious*, the usual duration of life is still less than in the latter class of malformation. Of 22 such cases, in which the patients survived for a longer or shorter period after birth, 9 died before the age of three months, 3 between three and six months, 3 between six and twelve months, 3 between twelve months and two years, 3 lived to the ages of nine or ten, and 1 of twelve years. Dr. Hare's patient attained the age of nine months, and my own of eleven months and two weeks. In the case reported by Dr. Ramsbotham as one of absence of the pulmonary artery, but in which that vessel exists though only in a rudimentary condition, the patient died when sixteen years old.

Where the arrest of development is still more complete, so that the *heart consists of only one ventricle with one or two auricles*, the period for which the patients survive is usually very limited : but it is very remarkable that four persons who presented this condition attained the ages of eleven, sixteen, twenty-three, and twenty-four years. Dr. Hale's patient lived nineteen weeks. Of five cases in which the heart is said to have consisted only of a single auricle and ventricle, the infants survived seventy-eight hours, seventy-nine hours, seven days, and, in two cases, three days ; but in four cases in which the arrest of development was less complete, the patients lived ten days, ten weeks, four months, and ten and a half-months. I have not thought it necessary, in speaking of the age of patients presenting these extreme forms of malformation, to allude to the cases of Pozzi and Lanzoni, for, as previously stated, they are too imperfectly reported for their nature to be distinctly understood. Neither can I regard the statement here given of the duration of life in the published cases, as showing the ordinary viability of persons labouring under such malformations. The circumstance of any one surviving for several years, with a heart which was found to present any of these conditions, would be regarded as so remarkable as to secure the case being placed on record ; whereas it is probable that similar malformations may have been frequently met with in infants, without attracting much attention. The inference to be drawn from the facts is rather that the curtailment of life generally bears reference to the degree of impediment to the circulation of the blood; but that there is scarcely any amount of arrest of development which is not compatible with the occasional prolongation of life for some years.

Where an *abnormal septum exists in the right ventricle*, the duration of life bears reference to the degree of obstruction which is occasioned, and the effects correspond very closely with those which result from an impediment at the pulmonic orifice. Thus in the cases in which, in addition to the obstruction caused by the septum, there was a communication between the two ventricles, the patients survived to the ages of nine, ten, fourteen, twenty, and twenty-two years, and the subject of my first case of the kind died at the age of fifteen. In these instances the pulmonary orifice also was contracted, though the impediment thus created was much less than that caused by the supernumerary septum. In Mr. Clark's case the openings through the septum were very small but the pulmonic orifice was not contracted, and the boy lived to the age of nineteen. In Dr. Thompson's case the septal obstruction was moderate, and the pulmonary orifice was enlarged, and the patient died at the age of thirty-eight. In Mr. Hutchinson's patient the obstruction was greater than in any of the others and the heart was otherwise very imperfectly developed, yet she survived to the age of twelve. In my own case, in which the heart was naturally formed except for the existence of the septum, the patient died at the age of five years of hæmorrhage from the throat or stomach during an attack of scarlatina; and M. Claude Bernard's patient, who presented a similar defect, attained the age of fifty-six. The congenital origin of the disease may, however, be disputed in this case, indeed the obstruction is supposed by the author to have been the result of endocarditis, occurring during an attack of acute rheumatism.

The *transposition of the main arteries* appears to be a form of malformation which is incompatible with the maintenance of life for any considerable period after birth. Of 16 cases of this description, 3 proved fatal within the first week, 1 in the second, and 1 in the third week; 1 at the sixth week; 2 at two months; 2 at ten weeks; 1 at five months; 1 at seven months, and 1 at ten months; and 3 others at two years and six months, two years and seven months, and two years and nine months. In the case of Mr. Gamage, in which the viscera of the body generally were transposed, the infant lived fifteen weeks. In that reported by Dr. Hess and myself, in which there were other defects in the conformation of the heart, the child survived eight months. The existence of defect in the septum of the ventricles, though of rare occurrence in this class of cases, appears, as might be expected, to be favourable to the prolongation of life. Of four such cases, 3 of the patients survived from seven months and eight days to two years and nine months. The closure of the ductus arteriosus, when the septum of the ventricles is entire, would, on the contrary, seem to add so greatly to the difficulty in transmitting the blood to the lungs, as to be scarcely compatible with the maintenance of life. In two cases, however, in which it is stated that this condition existed and the only communication between the two sides of the heart was through the foramen ovale, the patients died at the ages of fifteen weeks and two and a-half years.

The duration of life in the form of malformation in which *the aorta distal to the left subclavian artery is contracted or impervious, and the descending aorta is wholly or chiefly supplied through the pulmonary artery,* is generally very limited. In the two cases which occurred to Sir Astley Cooper, the infants lived two days, and eight months ; Dr. Rees' patient survived ten weeks. In the more aggravated form of this malformation, described by Steidele, the infant died shortly after birth. In M. Gibert's case the child lived twelve days, and the subject of the case related by Dr. Greig, was still-born. It is probable, that in cases of this description the ready outlet for the blood from the pulmonary artery into the abdominal aorta, prevents the free entrance of blood into the lungs, and so interferes with the full expansion of those organs.

When the heart is well formed, its *malposition* within the thorax, is not necessarily productive of such serious inconvenience as to interfere with the duration of life. In Dr. Sampson's case the patient was thirty years of age; in

Dr. Baillie's, nearly forty ; and in M. Meckel's it would appear from the plate, that the subject in whom the malformation was found must have been an adult. Instances are, indeed, on record in which the heart with the other viscera of the body have been transposed, in persons who survived to advanced age and had never presented any evidence of embarrassment of the circulation. The subject of the case described by M. Mery had been a soldier and died at seventy-two years of age ; and a still more remarkable instance is mentioned by M. Bosc, in which the patient lived to the age of eighty-four. When the heart is situated in the abdomen, life also may be much prolonged. The patient mentioned by Deschamps, in whom the heart occupied the position of the left kidney, was a soldier who had served for many years in the army. Where, on the other hand, the heart occupies a position entirely external to the cavity of the chest, there is most generally some serious defect in the conformation of the organ or other viscera of the body, so that life is usually maintained only for a very limited period. In Mr. Sidney Jones' case, in which the heart was situated entirely external to the thorax, the infant only lived thirteen hours ; but, in the case mentioned by Dr. O'Bryan, the organ was situated in part externally, and the child survived three months.

The *absence of the pericardium* does not appear to affect the functions of the heart or to interfere with the duration of life, though the organ, under such circumstances, very generally contracts adhesions to the adjacent parts. All the cases quoted, occurred in persons who had attained adult or middle age, and none of them were known to have manifested during life, any symptoms of disorder of the heart or circulation.

The *malformations of the valves* vary in their effects according to the nature of the irregularity. When the number of the segments is defective, and especially when the whole of them are united together, some obstruction is generally occasioned, and the valves are apt to become the seat of subsequent disease, and life is usually more or less curtailed. I have, however, occasionally seen only two valves at the aortic orifice in persons who have died in advanced life, and frequently in middle age.

When, on the contrary, the number is in excess, no inconvenience may result, and life may be maintained to the full period. I have figured a specimen in which there were four valves to the pulmonary artery, taken from a woman seventy-five years of age.

The causes of death in cases of malformation of the heart are—

1st. Cerebral disturbance resulting from the defective aëration of the blood and congestion of the brain.

2ndly. Imperfect expansion, collapse and engorgement of the lungs.

3rdly. Effusion into the cellular tissue and serous sacs from failure of the power of the heart, or recent disease superinduced on the original cardiac defect.

4thly. Exhaustion from the imperfect performance of the respiratory functions and the circulation of blood in great part venous.

5thly. Other diseases predisposed to by the defective conformation of the heart ; as apoplexy or paralysis from engorgement or softening of the brain, or extravasation of blood ; congestion or inflammation of the lungs, croup, bronchitis, pneumonia, pulmonary apoplexy and hæmoptysis, pleurisy, &c. ; disorder of the digestive organs, vomiting, diarrhœa, jaundice, &c. ; renal and tuberculous affections, &c., with other diseases occurring accidentally.

Of these different causes the two first are by far the most frequent and especially in children in which the heart is very imperfect and life is therefore only prolonged for a very limited period. Serious dropsical affections less frequently occur than the degree of obstruction to the circulation would lead us to expect. Gradual exhaustion from imperfect nutrition and disorder of the digestive organs, are occasionally the causes of death both in infants and older subjects.

I have already mentioned that cerebral and pulmonary diseases and hæmoptysis are frequently fatal when the patients survive several years, and death also occasionally occurs from tuberculous affections of the lungs, especially when life is maintained to the age of ten or fifteen. In a patient of my own, who lived to the age of twenty,[1] in whom the pulmonary artery was greatly contracted and the foramen ovale largely open, and in a case related by Dr. Leared,[2] in which the patient died at the age of eight and presented similar defects, the lungs were found tuberculous. In the young woman whose case was reported by Dr. Ramsbotham,[3] as one of absence of the pulmonary artery with compensatory branches from the aorta, death occurred from phthisis ; and that disease was also partly the cause of death, in the boy whose case is related by Dr. Shearman,[4] in whom the pulmonary artery was obliterated. Death ensued from the same cause in another boy, mentioned by Dr. Cheevers[5] of Boston, in whom the pulmonary artery was nearly impervious, the septum of the ventricles imperfect, and the foramen ovale and ductus arteriosus open. In cases related by Gregory,[6] Bertody and Dunglisson,[7] Gintrac,[8] and Louis,[9] in persons, aged respectively eighteen, twenty-one, twenty-one, and twenty-five, in whom the pulmonary artery was contracted and the septum of the ventricles defective, the lungs were also tuberculous.

I have been the more particular in alluding to these cases as they are opposed to the assertion of Rokitansky that tuberculosis does not " coexist with congenital vices of formation of the heart, or great arterial trunks, which, with their complications, result in venosity and cyanosis,"[10] and that " all cyanoses, or rather all forms of disease of the heart, vessels or lungs, inducing cyanosis of various kinds and degrees, are incompatible with

[1] Case VIII., p. 83, supra.   [2] Dublin Journal, N. S., vol. 10, 1850, p. 223.

[3] Med. and Phys. Jour., vol. 61, (N. S., vol. 6), p. 548. In a female, 16 years of age.

[4] Prov. Med. and Surg. Jour., 1845, p. 484. In a female of 9 years of age.

[5] New England Jour. of Med. and Surg., vol. 10, 1821, (N. S., vol. 5), p. 217. In a boy 13½ years old.

[6] Med. Chir. Trans., vol. 11, 1820, p. 296.

[7] Phil. Med. Ex., 1845, quoted in Dublin Jour., vol. 28, 1845, p. 300.

[8] Sur la Cyanose, obs. 45.

[9] Arch. Gén. dé Méd., 2me serie, t. 3, 1823, obs. 9, and Memoires et Recherches Anatomico-pathologiques, 1826, obs. 10, p. 313.

[10] Pathological Anatomy, Sydenham Society's translation, vol. 1, p. 316.

tuberculosis, against which cyanosis affords a complete protection."[1]

In the cases which I have referred to, the cyanosis existed to a marked degree in six, but was only occasionally noticed in three. In most of them, it was observed at or shortly after birth and continued throughout life. In all the cases but a small portion of blood could have been submitted to the influence of the air in the lungs, the freest intermixture of the currents must have existed, and the blood circulating in the systemic vessels must have been to a great extent venous. Yet this condition did not prevent the occurrence of tuberculosis. On the contrary, active tuberculous disease was present in every case, there being either miliary tubercles, softened tubercle, or cavities in the lungs. As these cases constituted nine, or 16·07 per cent. of fifty-six, in which the patients, with different forms of malformation, survived the age of eight, it might even be supposed that tuberculous affections are more common in persons with defects in the conformation of the heart than in the population at large.[2] This would, however, probably be carrying the inference too far. It is possible that the venous condition of the blood may, as supposed by Laennec, be in some degree opposed to the occurrence of tuberculous affections, but this opposition certainly in no degree amounts to an incompatibility, as asserted by Rokitansky. Every medical man of much experience has also met with cases in which tuberculosis has occurred in persons long subject to chronic bronchitis and asthma. In the case of malformation related by M. M. Aran and Deguise,[3] the patient died of disease of the hip.

DIAGNOSIS.

The detection of the existence of malformation of the heart, in ordinary cases, when the patient is seen in early life, can

---

[1] Pathological Anatomy, Sydenham Society's translation, vol. 4, p. 251.

[2] From the Registrar-General's Report for 1854, it appears that the cases of consumption constituted only 9·1 per cent. of the total number of deaths in England and Wales.

[3] Lancet, 1844 ; and Bullet. de la Soc. Anat., 1842, &c.

scarcely present any difficulty. The statement that palpitation, dyspnœa, and more or less cyanosis, had existed since birth, or shortly after, and the evidences of obstructed circulation at the time of examination, render the case sufficiently clear. M. Louis, indeed, regards the occurrence of "suffocative attacks brought on by the slightest cause, often periodic, and always very frequent, and accompanied or followed by syncope, and with or without the blue discoloration of the body generally," as pathognomonic of communications between the right and left cavities of the heart; and the cyanotic discoloration, when present can scarcely be mistaken. But the ordinary symptoms may be absent or may exist only to a slight degree, or the patient may not be seen till after he has attained the age of puberty or manhood and there may be no satisfactory history of his previous state of health to aid the diagnosis. Though, in cases of this kind, if the patients had been under medical care, it is quite possible that sufficiently characteristic signs might have been observed, we are sometimes assured by the patient and his friends that he had enjoyed good health, had been capable of following a laborious occupation, and had presented nothing unusual in his appearance, until shortly before the time at which he falls under our notice. In such cases, then, it may be extremely difficult to decide whether the patient labours under some form of malformation, or under ordinary disease of the heart; and the differential diagnosis can only be effected by a careful examination and analysis of the general symptoms and physical signs.

In all cases, also, the detection of the precise form of malformation must be a task of considerable difficulty, and in some instances entirely impracticable. Where an infant suffers from great difficulty of breathing and palpitation, and is intensely and constantly cyanosed, at or immediately after birth, it may be inferred that it labours under some serious malformation occasioning great obstruction to the circulation of the blood, as obliteration or great contraction of the pulmonic orifice, or transposition of the aorta and pulmonary artery. On the contrary, when the symptoms do not manifest themselves at so early a period, and are less constant and intense, there is probably only some slighter malformation, as a moderate amount of contraction at the pulmonary orifice. Of 153 cases of various forms of decided and important malformation, of which I have collected notes, in 74 there existed more or less contraction of the orifice of the pulmonary artery or other sources of obstruction to the exit of the blood from the right ventricle, and in 25 others the orifice or trunk of the vessel was obliterated. In those patients who survived the age of twelve, the entrance of the blood into the pulmonary artery was interfered with in a much larger proportion of cases, or in 32 out of 39; so that, in any given case of malformation, especially after the age of fifteen, the probability is that the pulmonary artery is contracted. If this be the case, a loud systolic murmur will be heard in the præcordial region, and most intensely at the level of the nipple and between that body and the sternum. It will be audible very distinctly in the course of the pulmonary artery, or from the base of the heart towards the middle of the left clavicle; and less distinctly in the course of the aorta, or at the upper part and right side of the sternum. If the pulmonic orifice be permanently open as is often the case, especially where the whole of the valves are united, there may also be a diastolic murmur; but, from the very small size of the aperture in most instances, the regurgitant current is probably generally too slight to generate a distinct murmur. Most usually with considerable contraction of the pulmonary orifice, the septum of the ventricles is defective, and the aorta derives its supply of blood from both ventricles; and, if so, a systolic murmur may probably be produced by the meeting of the two columns of blood in the ascending aorta, which may modify the signs observed. Generally, in such cases, the aorta is unusually large, and, from the powerful re-action on the valves during the diastole of the heart, a loud ringing second sound is heard on listening at the upper part of the sternum. With these signs there will also be perceived those of hypertrophy and dilatation of the right ventricle and auricle, and frequently a distinct jugular pulsation will be observed. The heart being much increased in size and its walls hypertrophied, the dull space will be extended beyond its usual limits, especially towards the right side. From the yielding of the parietes in early life, the præcordia is also generally prominent. The impulse of the heart is usually powerful, and frequently a distinct purring tremor may be felt over the situation of the pulmonic orifice. The pulse is generally quick, small, and weak. It has been thought that, in cases of obstruction at the right side of the heart, the patient is disposed to let the head hang down so as to compress the chest, rather than to adopt the upright position, which we most frequently see selected by patients with disease of the left orifices; but I have seen patients with aortic disease hang themselves completely over the side of the bed, so that this rule does not certainly apply.

If the evidence of obstruction at the pulmonic orifice be tolerably conclusive, we may safely infer there is either a deficiency in the septum of the ventricles, or a patent foramen ovale, for one or other of these defects almost invariably co-exists with that condition. An aperture in the septum of the ventricles, without other malformation, would probably be attended by a murmur, caused by the flow of blood through the abnormal opening from the left ventricle into the right ventricle or auricle. The detection, therefore, of a systolic murmur at the base of the heart, without signs of obstruction at the aortic or pulmonic orifice, might lead to a suspicion that such a communication existed. This surmise would be strengthened if the murmur were not propagated in the course of the pulmonary artery or aorta; and especially if the patient were long under notice, and constantly presented the sign, without other evidence of cardiac disease or defect; and without having had any disease or accident during life which could probably have produced such a change in the heart as would be likely to be attended by a permanent murmur.

I do not know that there are any means of detecting the open state of the foramen ovale; and there are also other malformations of the heart, such as transposition of the aorta and pulmonary artery, which could not be at all diagnosed during life.

In some cases, as where the ductus arteriosus or foramen ovale remains open, the diagnosis may be aided by ascertaining whether the infant has been born prematurely or at the full period.

It has already been mentioned that the malformations of the valves do not necessarily entail any interference with the functions of the heart. When they lead to disease of the organ, the symptoms and physical signs will be those of valvular disease dependant on any other cause. I believe that when a patient in early or adult life labours under symptoms of valvular disease, more especially at the aortic orifice, without having previously sustained any severe injury or strain, and without having had any serious rheumatic attack, we shall generally be correct in inferring that the valves are malformed.

MEDICAL TREATMENT.

The medical treatment in cases of malformation of the heart must consist, first, in the hygienic management of the patient, so as to maintain the circulation, and give tone to the general system; secondly, in the avoidance of the various causes which may aggravate the existing defects in the conformation of the heart, or give rise to secondary disease in other organs; and, thirdly, in the relief of the urgent symptoms when they arise.

1st. The surface should be carefully protected against cold, so as to economize the scanty power of generating heat, and this may be accomplished by warm clothing, and especially by wearing flannel, or some other woollen material, or silk, next the skin. The patient should reside in a warm situation if practicable, and the room which he occupies should be maintained at an agreeable and equable temperature. His strength should be upheld by nutritious food, and a moderate quantity of stimulus, malt liquor or wine, should be allowed. The secretions should be regulated by gentle exercise, in the nurse's arms if the patient be an infant, or in a carriage if an older person; and when the weather is suitable he should frequently be in the open air. The cutaneous functions, which may greatly compensate for the defective aëration of the blood in the lungs, should be promoted by warm or tepid bathing or ablution, followed by friction of the surface.

2ndly. The patient should be kept quiet and undue excitement of mind and fatigue of body should be avoided. Sudden exposure to cold and damp should be specially guarded against, lest the patient should become the subject of any form of pulmonary disease which would greatly aggravate the general congestion; or of rheumatism, which would almost certainly implicate the heart. Care should also be exercised that the food which is taken should be easily digestible, and that the stomach should not be overloaded or the secretions checked, as neglect of these circumstances would be very likely to bring on attacks of dyspnœa or convulsions. Over-excitement of the brain should be especially guarded against.

3rdly. For the relief of the paroxysms when they occur, the first indication is to ascertain the cause by which they have been induced. If undue exertion of body or excitement of mind have caused the attack, it will probably subside on entire rest. If the stomach have been overloaded or indigestible food have been taken, an emetic or a mild aperient, may be given, and if the symptoms do not afterwards subside, the patient may be treated by antispasmodics—the warm bath, ether, ammonia, &c and anodynes.

In most cases of malformation the patients labour under dyspeptic symptoms, the bowels are generally torpid, and the attacks are often occasioned or aggravated by flatulency. For the relief of these symptoms small doses of hydragyrum cum cretâ, with rhubarb, soda or magnesia, and followed by bitter tonics, are very beneficial. When there is much palpitation or pain in the region of the heart, hydrocyanic acid, hyoscyamus, and opiates are applicable. The Dover's powder is especially useful, not only by acting as a mild anodyne, but also by promoting diaphresis. The convulsive attacks to which cyanotic persons are subject, are often relieved by the application of a few leeches to the temples or behind the ears, and in children which are teething the pressure of the gums may be removed by lancing. From, however, the scanty aëration of the blood and its consequent deficiency in fibrine, and from the excessive congestion of all parts of the system, the flow of blood either from leech-bites or incisions is apt to be excessive, and in some cases

I have seen dangerous hæmorrhage. Great care should therefore be practised, in having recourse to these means, that the loss of blood shall not exceed the required amount.

By the course of management which has been mentioned in the slighter forms of malformation, life may occasionally be prolonged for several years, and in some instances a considerable amount of constitutional vigour may be enjoyed; but such cases are exceptional and only occur under the most favourable circumstances. In the more serious deviations from the natural conformation of the heart, which constitute the majority of the cases, the maintenance of life is unavoidably limited to a few days, weeks, or months, and the benefit to be derived from medicine is confined to affording some alleviation to the sufferings of the patient.

LONDON : RICHARD BARRETT, PRINTER, MARK LANE.

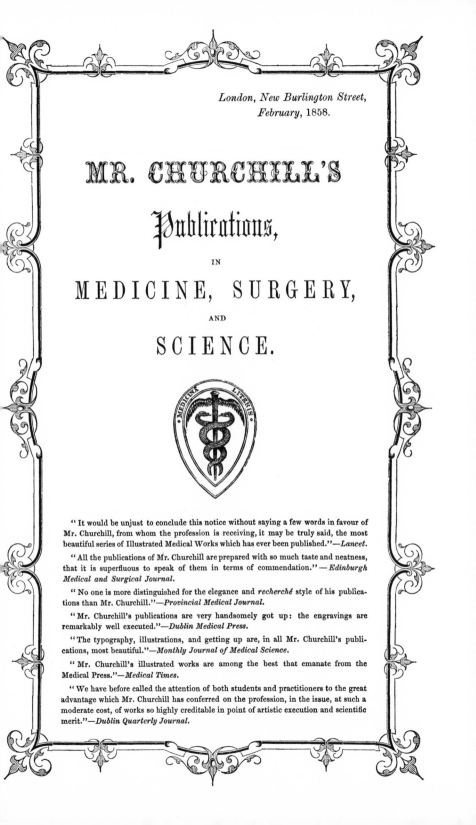

London, New Burlington Street,
February, 1858.

MR. CHURCHILL'S

Publications,

IN

MEDICINE, SURGERY,

AND

SCIENCE.

"It would be unjust to conclude this notice without saying a few words in favour of Mr. Churchill, from whom the profession is receiving, it may be truly said, the most beautiful series of Illustrated Medical Works which has ever been published."—*Lancet.*

"All the publications of Mr. Churchill are prepared with so much taste and neatness, that it is superfluous to speak of them in terms of commendation." — *Edinburgh Medical and Surgical Journal.*

"No one is more distinguished for the elegance and *recherché* style of his publications than Mr. Churchill."—*Provincial Medical Journal.*

"Mr. Churchill's publications are very handsomely got up: the engravings are remarkably well executed."—*Dublin Medical Press.*

"The typography, illustrations, and getting up are, in all Mr. Churchill's publications, most beautiful."—*Monthly Journal of Medical Science.*

"Mr. Churchill's illustrated works are among the best that emanate from the Medical Press."—*Medical Times.*

"We have before called the attention of both students and practitioners to the great advantage which Mr. Churchill has conferred on the profession, in the issue, at such a moderate cost, of works so highly creditable in point of artistic execution and scientific merit."—*Dublin Quarterly Journal.*

Mr. Churchill is the Publisher of the following Periodicals, offering to Authors a wide extent of Literary Announcement, and a Medium of Advertisement, addressed to all Classes of the Profession. Communications, Books for Review, addressed to the respective Editors, are received and duly forwarded by Mr. Churchill.

THE BRITISH AND FOREIGN MEDICO-CHIRURGICAL REVIEW;

OR,

QUARTERLY JOURNAL OF PRACTICAL MEDICINE.

Price Six Shillings. Nos. I. to XLI.

THE QUARTERLY JOURNAL OF MICROSCOPICAL SCIENCE.

Edited by Edwin Lankester, M.D., F.R.S., F.L.S., and George Busk, F.R.C.S.E., F.R.S., F.L.S. Price 4s. Nos. I. to XXII.

THE MEDICAL TIMES AND GAZETTE.

Published Weekly, price Sevenpence, or Stamped, Eightpence.
Annual Subscription, £1.10s., or Stamped, £1. 14s. 8d., and regularly forwarded to all parts of the Kingdom.

The Medical Times and Gazette is favoured with an amount of Literary and Scientific support which enables it to reflect fully the progress of Medical Science, and insure for it a character, an influence, and a circulation possessed at the present time by no Medical Periodical.

THE HALF-YEARLY ABSTRACT OF THE MEDICAL SCIENCES.

Being a Digest of the Contents of the principal British and Continental Medical Works; together with a Critical Report of the Progress of Medicine and the Collateral Sciences. Edited by W. H. Ranking, M.D., Cantab., and C. B. Radcliffe, M.D., Lond. Post 8vo. cloth, 6s. 6d. Vols. I. to XXVI.

THE JOURNAL OF PSYCHOLOGICAL MEDICINE AND MENTAL PATHOLOGY.

Being a Quarterly Review of Medical Jurisprudence and Insanity. Edited by Forbes Winslow, M.D. Price 3s. 6d. Nos. I. to IX. *New Series.*

THE PHARMACEUTICAL JOURNAL.

EDITED BY JACOB BELL, F.L.S., M.R.I.

Published Monthly, price One Shilling.

*** Vols. I. to XV., bound in cloth, price 12s. 6d. each.

THE DUBLIN MEDICAL PRESS.

Published Weekly, Stamped, price Sixpence, free to any part of the Empire.

THE LONDON AND PROVINCIAL MEDICAL DIRECTORY.

Published Annually. 12mo. cloth, 8s. 6d.

A CLASSIFIED INDEX

TO

MR. CHURCHILL'S CATALOGUE.

CLASSIFIED INDEX.

DR. ACLAND.

MEMOIR ON THE CHOLERA AT OXFORD IN THE YEAR
1854; with Considerations suggested by the Epidemic. 4to. cloth, with Maps, 12s.

MR. ACTON, M.R.C.S.
I.

THE FUNCTIONS AND DISORDERS OF THE REPRODUC-
TIVE ORGANS IN YOUTH, IN ADULT AGE, AND IN ADVANCED
LIFE. Considered in their Physiological, Social, and Psychological Relations. Second
Edition. 8vo. cloth, 7s.

II.

PROSTITUTION : Considered in its Moral, Social, and Sanitary Bearings,
with a View to its Amelioration and Regulation. 8vo. cloth, 10s. 6d.

III.

A PRACTICAL TREATISE ON DISEASES OF THE URINARY
AND GENERATIVE ORGANS OF BOTH SEXES, INCLUDING SYPHILIS.
Second Edition. 8vo. cloth, 20s.

DR. WILLIAM ADDISON, F.R.S.
I.

CELL THERAPEUTICS. 8vo. cloth, 4s.

II.

ON HEALTHY AND DISEASED STRUCTURE, AND THE TRUE
PRINCIPLES OF TREATMENT FOR THE CURE OF DISEASE, ESPECIALLY CONSUMPTION
AND SCROFULA, founded on MICROSCOPICAL ANALYSIS. 8vo. cloth, 12s.

DR. ALEXANDER, F.R.C.S. BY EXAM.

RHEUMATISM : its Nature, Causes, and Cure.
GOUT : its Nature, Causes, Cure, and Prevention.
Post 8vo. cloth, 7s. 6d.

MR. ANDERSON, F.R.C.S.

THE CAUSES, SYMPTOMS, & TREATMENT OF ECCENTRIC
NERVOUS AFFECTIONS. 8vo. cloth, 5s.

THE ANATOMICAL REMEMBRANCER; OR, COMPLETE
POCKET ANATOMIST. Fifth Edition, carefully Revised. 32mo. cloth, 3s. 6d.

DR. JAMES ARNOTT.
I.

ON THE REMEDIAL AGENCY OF A LOCAL ANÆSTHENIC
OR BENUMBING TEMPERATURE, in various painful and inflammatory Diseases.
8vo. cloth, 4s. 6d.

II.

ON INDIGESTION ; its Pathology and its Treatment, by the Local
Application of Uniform and Continuous Heat and Moisture. With an Account of an
improved Mode of applying Heat and Moisture in Irritative and Inflammatory Diseases.
With a Plate. 8vo. 5s.

III.

PRACTICAL ILLUSTRATIONS OF THE TREATMENT OF
OBSTRUCTIONS IN THE URETHRA, AND OTHER CANALS, BY THE
DILATATION OF FLUID PRESSURE. 8vo. boards, 3s.

MR. F. A. ABEL, F.C.S., & MR. C. L. BLOXAM.

HANDBOOK OF CHEMISTRY: THEORETICAL, PRACTICAL, AND TECHNICAL. 8vo. cloth, 15s.

DR. ADAMS, A.M.

A TREATISE ON RHEUMATIC GOUT; OR, CHRONIC RHEUMATIC ARTHRITIS. 8vo. cloth, with a Quarto Atlas of Plates, 21s.

DR. ADDISON.

ON THE CONSTITUTIONAL AND LOCAL EFFECTS OF DISEASE OF THE SUPRA-RENAL CAPSULES. 4to. cloth. Coloured Plates, 21s.

MR. T. J. ASHTON.

ON THE DISEASES, INJURIES, AND MALFORMATIONS OF THE RECTUM AND ANUS. Second Edition. 8vo. cloth, 8s.

MR. ATKINSON.

MEDICAL BIBLIOGRAPHY. Vol. I. Royal 8vo. 16s.

DR. WILLIAM BALY, F.R.S., & DR. WILLIAM W. GULL.

REPORTS ON EPIDEMIC CHOLERA; its Cause and Mode of Diffusion, Morbid Anatomy, Pathology and Treatment. Drawn up at the desire of the Cholera Committee of the Royal College of Physicians. With Maps, 8vo. cloth, 16s.

DR. BARLOW.

A MANUAL OF THE PRACTICE OF MEDICINE. Fcap. 8vo. cloth, 12s. 6d.

DR. BARNES.

THE PHYSIOLOGY AND TREATMENT OF PLACENTA PRÆVIA; being the Lettsomian Lectures on Midwifery for 1857. Post 8vo. cloth, 6s.

DR. BASCOME.

A HISTORY OF EPIDEMIC PESTILENCES, FROM THE EARLIEST AGES. 8vo. cloth, 8s.

MR. BATEMAN.

MAGNACOPIA: A Practical Library of Profitable Knowledge, communicating the general Minutiæ of Chemical and Pharmaceutic Routine, together with the generality of Secret Forms of Preparations; including Concentrated Solutions of Camphor and Copaiba in Water, Mineral Succedaneum, Marmoratum, Silicia, Terro-Metallicum, Pharmaceutic Condensions, Prismatic Crystallization, Crystallized Aromatic Salt of Vinegar, Spa Waters; newly-invented Writing Fluids; Etching on Steel or Iron; with an extensive Variety of et cætera. Third Edition. 18mo. 6s.

DR. BEALE.

I.

HOW TO WORK WITH THE MICROSCOPE. Crown 8vo. cloth, 5s.

II.

THE MICROSCOPE, AND ITS APPLICATION TO CLINICAL MEDICINE. With 232 Engravings on Wood. Post 8vo. cloth, 10s. 6d.

III.

ON THE ANATOMY OF THE LIVER. Illustrated with 66 Photographs of the Author's Drawings. 8vo. cloth, 6s. 6d.

MR. LIONEL J. BEALE, M.R.C.S.

I.

THE LAWS OF HEALTH IN THEIR RELATIONS TO MIND AND BODY. A Series of Letters from an Old Practitioner to a Patient. Post 8vo. cloth, 7s. 6d.

II.

HEALTH AND DISEASE, IN CONNECTION WITH THE GENERAL PRINCIPLES OF HYGIENE. Fcap. 8vo., 2s. 6d.

DR. BARCLAY.

A MANUAL OF MEDICAL DIAGNOSIS. Fcap. 8vo. cloth, 8s. 6d.

MR. BEASLEY.

I.

THE BOOK OF PRESCRIPTIONS; containing 2900 Prescriptions. Collected from the Practice of the most eminent Physicians and Surgeons, English and Foreign. 24mo. cloth, 6s.

II.

THE DRUGGISTS' GENERAL RECEIPT-BOOK: comprising a copious Veterinary Formulary and Table of Veterinary Materia Medica; Patent and Proprietary Medicines, Druggists' Nostrums, &c.; Perfumery, Skin Cosmetics, Hair Cosmetics, and Teeth Cosmetics; Beverages, Dietetic Articles, and Condiments; Trade Chemicals, Miscellaneous Preparations and Compounds used in the Arts, &c.; with useful Memoranda and Tables. Fourth Edition. 24mo. cloth, 6s.

III.

THE POCKET FORMULARY AND SYNOPSIS OF THE BRITISH AND FOREIGN PHARMACOPŒIAS; comprising standard and approved Formulæ for the Preparations and Compounds employed in Medical Practice. Sixth Edition, corrected and enlarged. 24mo. cloth, 6s.

DR. O'B. BELLINGHAM.

ON ANEURISM, AND ITS TREATMENT BY COMPRESSION. 12mo. cloth, 4s.

DR. HENRY BENNET.

I.

A PRACTICAL TREATISE ON INFLAMMATION AND OTHER DISEASES OF THE UTERUS. Third Edition, revised, with Additions. 8vo. cloth, 12s. 6d.

II.

A REVIEW OF THE PRESENT STATE OF UTERINE PATHOLOGY. 8vo. cloth, 4s.

DR. BILLING, F.R.S.

I.

ON DISEASES OF THE LUNGS AND HEART. 8vo. cloth, 6s.

II.

FIRST PRINCIPLES OF MEDICINE. Fifth Edition, Revised and Improved. 8vo. 10s. 6d.

MR. HENRY HEATHER BIGG.

ARTIFICIAL LIMBS; THEIR CONSTRUCTION AND APPLI-
CATION. With Engravings on Wood. 8vo. cloth, 3s.

MR. P. HINCKES BIRD, F.R.C.S.

PRACTICAL TREATISE ON THE DISEASES OF CHILDREN
AND INFANTS AT THE BREAST. Translated from the French of M. BOUCHUT,
with Notes and Additions. 8vo. cloth. 20s.

DR. GOLDING BIRD, F.R.S.

I.

URINARY DEPOSITS; THEIR DIAGNOSIS, PATHOLOGY,
AND THERAPEUTICAL INDICATIONS. With Engravings on Wood. Fifth
Edition. Post 8vo. cloth, 10s. 6d.

II.

ELEMENTS OF NATURAL PHILOSOPHY; being an Experimental
Introduction to the Study of the Physical Sciences. Illustrated with numerous Engrav-
ings on Wood. Fourth Edition. By GOLDING BIRD, M.D., F.R.S., and CHARLES
BROOKE, M.B. Cantab., F.R.S. Fcap. 8vo. cloth, 12s. 6d.

MR. JAMES BIRD.

VEGETABLE CHARCOAL: its MEDICINAL and ECONOMIC PRO-
PERTIES; with Practical Remarks on its Use in Chronic Affections of the Stomach
and Bowels. Second Edition, 8vo. cloth, 3s. 6d.

MR. BISHOP, F.R.S.

I.

ON DEFORMITIES OF THE HUMAN BODY, their Pathology
and Treatment. With Engravings on Wood. 8vo. cloth, 10s.

II.

ON ARTICULATE SOUNDS, AND ON THE CAUSES AND
CURE OF IMPEDIMENTS OF SPEECH. 8vo. cloth, 4s.

III.

LETTSOMIAN LECTURES ON THE PHYSICAL CONSTI-
TUTION, DISEASES AND FRACTURES OF BONES. Post 8vo., 2s. 6d.

DR. BLAKISTON, F.R.S.

PRACTICAL OBSERVATIONS ON CERTAIN DISEASES OF
THE CHEST; and on the Principles of Auscultation. 8vo. cloth, 12s.

DR. JOHN W. F. BLUNDELL.

MEDICINA MECHANICA; or, the Theory and Practice of Active and
Passive Exercises and Manipulations in the Cure of Chronic Disease. Post 8vo. cloth, 6s.

MR. WALTER BLUNDELL.

PAINLESS TOOTH-EXTRACTION WITHOUT CHLOROFORM;
with Observations on Local Anæsthesia by Congelation in General Surgery. Second
Edition, 2s. 6d. cloth. Illustrated on Wood and Stone.

MR. JOHN E. BOWMAN.

I.

PRACTICAL CHEMISTRY, including Analysis. With numerous Illustrations on Wood. Third Edition. Foolscap 8vo. cloth, 6s. 6d.

II.

MEDICAL CHEMISTRY; with Illustrations on Wood. Third Edition. Fcap. 8vo. cloth, 6s. 6d.

DR. BRINTON.

THE SYMPTOMS, PATHOLOGY, AND TREATMENT OF ULCER OF THE STOMACH. Post 8vo. cloth, 5s.

DR. JAMES BRIGHT.

ON DISEASES OF THE CHEST AND AIR PASSAGES; with a Review of the several Climates recommended in these Affections. Second Edition. Post 8vo. cloth, 7s. 6d.

MR. ISAAC BAKER BROWN, F.R.C.S.

I.

ON SOME DISEASES OF WOMEN ADMITTING OF SURGICAL TREATMENT. With Plates, 8vo. cloth, 10s. 6d.

II.

ON SCARLATINA: its Nature and Treatment. Second Edition. Fcap. 8vo. cloth, 3s.

MR. BERNARD E. BRODHURST.

I.

ON LATERAL CURVATURE OF THE SPINE: its Pathology and Treatment. Post 8vo. cloth, with Plates, 3s.

II.

ON THE NATURE AND TREATMENT OF CLUBFOOT AND ANALOGOUS DISTORTIONS involving the TIBIO-TARSAL ARTICULATION. With Engravings on Wood. 8vo. cloth, 4s. 6d.

DR. BUDD, F.R.S.

I.

ON DISEASES OF THE LIVER. Illustrated with Coloured Plates and Engravings on Wood. Third Edition. 8vo. cloth, 16s.

II.

ON THE ORGANIC DISEASES AND FUNCTIONAL DISORDERS OF THE STOMACH. 8vo. cloth, 9s.

DR. BURGESS.

THE MEDICAL AND LEGAL RELATIONS OF MADNESS; showing a Cellular Theory of Mind, and of Nerve Force, and also of Vegetative Vital Force. 8vo. cloth, 9s.

DR. BURNETT.

I.

THE PHILOSOPHY OF SPIRITS IN RELATION TO MATTER. 8vo. cloth, 9s.

II.

INSANITY TESTED BY SCIENCE. 8vo. cloth, 5s.

DP BRYCE.

ENGLAND AND FRANCE BEFORE SEBASTOPOL, looked at
from a Medical Point of View.   8vo. cloth, 6s.

MR. ROBERT B. CARTER, M.R.C.S.

I.

ON THE INFLUENCE OF EDUCATION AND TRAINING
IN PREVENTING DISEASES OF THE NERVOUS SYSTEM. Fcap. 8vo., 6s.

II.

THE PATHOLOGY AND TREATMENT OF HYSTERIA. Post
8vo. cloth, 4s. 6d.

DR. CARPENTER, F.R.S.

I.

PRINCIPLES OF HUMAN PHYSIOLOGY. With numerous Illustrations on Steel and Wood. Fifth Edition.   8vo. cloth, 26s.

II.

PRINCIPLES OF COMPARATIVE PHYSIOLOGY. Illustrated
with 300 Engravings on Wood. Fourth Edition. 8vo. cloth, 24s.

III.

A MANUAL OF PHYSIOLOGY. With numerous Illustrations on
Steel and Wood. Third Edition. Fcap. 8vo. cloth, 12s. 6d.

IV.

THE MICROSCOPE AND ITS REVELATIONS. With nume-
rous Engravings on Wood. Second Edition. Fcap. 8vo. cloth, 12s. 6d.

DR. CHAMBERS.

DIGESTION AND ITS DERANGEMENTS. Post 8vo. cloth, 10s. 6d.

MR. H. T. CHAPMAN, F.R.C.S.

I.

THE TREATMENT OF OBSTINATE ULCERS AND CUTA-
NEOUS ERUPTIONS OF THE LEG WITHOUT CONFINEMENT. Second
Edition. Post 8vo. cloth, 3s. 6d.

II.

VARICOSE VEINS : their Nature, Consequences, and Treatment, Pallia-
tive and Curative. Post 8vo. cloth, 3s. 6d.

DR. G. C. CHILD.

ON INDIGESTION, AND CERTAIN BILIOUS DISORDERS
OFTEN CONJOINED WITH IT. Second Edition. 8vo. cloth, 6s.

MR. J. PATERSON CLARK, M.A.

THE ODONTALGIST; OR, HOW TO PRESERVE THE TEETH,
CURE TOOTHACHE, AND REGULATE DENTITION FROM INFANCY
TO AGE. With plates. Post 8vo. cloth, 5s.

DR. CONOLLY.

THE CONSTRUCTION AND GOVERNMENT OF LUNATIC
ASYLUMS AND HOSPITALS FOR THE INSANE. With Plans. Post 8vo. cloth, 6s.

LEWIS CORNARO.

SURE METHODS OF ATTAINING A LONG AND HEALTH-
FUL LIFE. Thirty-eighth Edition. 18mo., 1s.

MR. COOLEY.
COMPREHENSIVE SUPPLEMENT TO THE PHARMACOPŒIAS.

THE CYCLOPÆDIA OF PRACTICAL RECEIPTS, AND COL-
LATERAL INFORMATION IN THE ARTS, PROFESSIONS, MANU-
FACTURES, AND TRADES, INCLUDING MEDICINE, PHARMACY, AND
DOMESTIC ECONOMY; designed as a Compendious Book of Reference for the
Manufacturer, Tradesman, Amateur, and Heads of Families. Third and greatly
enlarged Edition, 8vo. cloth, 26s.

MR. BRANSBY B. COOPER, F.R.S.

LECTURES ON THE PRINCIPLES AND PRACTICE OF SUR-
GERY. 8vo. cloth, 21s.

MR. W. WHITE COOPER.

ON NEAR SIGHT, AGED SIGHT, IMPAIRED VISION,
AND THE MEANS OF ASSISTING SIGHT. With 31 Illustrations on Wood.
Second Edition. Fcap. 8vo. cloth, 7s. 6d.

MR. COOPER.

A DICTIONARY OF PRACTICAL SURGERY; comprehending all
the most interesting Improvements, from the Earliest Times down to the Present Period.
Seventh Edition. One very thick volume, 8vo., 1l. 10s.

SIR ASTLEY COOPER, BART., F.R.S.

ON THE STRUCTURE AND DISEASES OF THE TESTIS.
Illustrated with 24 highly finished Coloured Plates. Second Edition. Royal 4to.
Reduced from £3. 3s. *to* £1. 10s.

MR. HOLMES COOTE, F.R.C.S.

A REPORT ON SOME IMPORTANT POINTS IN THE
TREATMENT OF SYPHILIS. 8vo. cloth, 5s.

DR. COPEMAN.

RECORDS OF OBSTETRIC CONSULTATION PRACTICE;
and a TRANSLATION of BUSCH and MOSER on UTERINE HÆMORRHAGE;
with Notes and Cases. Post 8vo. cloth, 5s.

DR. COTTLE.

A MANUAL OF HUMAN PHYSIOLOGY FOR STUDENTS;

being a Condensation of the Subject, a Conservation of the Matter, and a Record of Facts and Principles up to the present Day. Fcap. 8vo., 5s.

DR. COTTON.

I.

ON CONSUMPTION: Its Nature, Symptoms, and Treatment. To

which Essay was awarded the Fothergillian Gold Medal of the Medical Society of London. Second Edition. 8vo. cloth, 8s.

II.

PHTHISIS AND THE STETHOSCOPE: a concise Practical Guide

to the Physical Diagnosis of Consumption. Foolscap 8vo. cloth, 3s. 6d.

MR. COULSON.

I.

ON DISEASES OF THE BLADDER AND PROSTATE GLAND.

The Fifth Edition, revised and enlarged. 8vo. cloth, 10s. 6d.

II.

ON LITHOTRITY AND LITHOTOMY; with Engravings on Wood.

8vo. cloth, 8s.

III.

ON DISEASES OF THE JOINTS. 8vo. *In the Press.*

DR. JOHN GREEN CROSSE, F.R.S.

CASES IN MIDWIFERY, arranged, with an Introduction and Remarks

by EDWARD COPEMAN, M.D., F.R.C.S. 8vo. cloth, 7s. 6d.

MR. CURLING, F.R.S.

I.

OBSERVATIONS ON DISEASES OF THE RECTUM. Second

Edition. 8vo. cloth, 5s.

II.

A PRACTICAL TREATISE ON DISEASES OF THE TESTIS,

SPERMATIC CORD, AND SCROTUM. Second Edition, with Additions. 8vo. cloth, 14s.

MR. JOHN DALRYMPLE, F.R.S., F.R.C.S.

PATHOLOGY OF THE HUMAN EYE. Complete in Nine Fasciculi:

imperial 4to., 20s. each; half-bound morocco, gilt tops, 9l. 15s.

DR. DAVEY.

I.

THE GANGLIONIC NERVOUS SYSTEM: its Structure, Functions,

and Diseases. 8vo. cloth, 9s.

II.

ON THE NATURE AND PROXIMATE CAUSE OF IN-

SANITY. Post 8vo. cloth, 3s.

DR. HERBERT DAVIES.

ON THE PHYSICAL DIAGNOSIS OF DISEASES OF THE LUNGS AND HEART. Second Edition. Post 8vo. cloth, 8s.

MR. DIXON.

A GUIDE TO THE PRACTICAL STUDY OF DISEASES OF THE EYE. Post 8vo. cloth, 8s. 6d.

DR. TOOGOOD DOWNING.

NEURALGIA: its various Forms, Pathology, and Treatment. THE JACKSONIAN PRIZE ESSAY FOR 1850. 8vo. cloth, 10s. 6d.

DR. DRUITT, F.R.C.S.

THE SURGEON'S VADE-MECUM; with numerous Engravings on Wood. Seventh Edition. Foolscap 8vo. cloth, 12s. 6d.

DR. JOHN C. EGAN.

SYPHILITIC DISEASES: THEIR PATHOLOGY, DIAGNOSIS, AND TREATMENT: including Experimental Researches on Inoculation, as a Differential Agent in Testing the Character of these Affections. 8vo. cloth, 9s.

SIR JAMES EYRE, M.D.

I.

THE STOMACH AND ITS DIFFICULTIES. Fourth Edition. Fcap. 8vo. cloth, 2s. 6d.

II.

PRACTICAL REMARKS ON SOME EXHAUSTING DISEASES. Second Edition. Post 8vo. cloth, 4s. 6d.

DR. FELL.

A TREATISE ON CANCER AND ITS TREATMENT. 8vo. cloth, 5s.

This work embraces an account of the Remedies, external and internal, employed by the Author; the mode of their Preparation and Application.

DR. FENWICK.

ON SCROFULA AND CONSUMPTION. Clergyman's Sore Throat, Catarrh, Croup, Bronchitis, Asthma. Fcap. 8vo., 2s. 6d.

MR. FERGUSSON, F.R.S.

A SYSTEM OF PRACTICAL SURGERY; with numerous Illustrations on Wood. Fourth Edition. Fcap. 8vo. cloth, 12s. 6d.

SIR JOHN FORBES, M.D., D.C.L. (OXON.), F.R.S.

NATURE AND ART IN THE CURE OF DISEASE. Second
Edition. Post 8vo. cloth, 6s.

DR. D. J. T. FRANCIS.

CHANGE OF CLIMATE; considered as a Remedy in Dyspeptic, Pulmonary, and other Chronic Affections; with an Account of the most Eligible Places of Residence for Invalids in Spain, Portugal, Algeria, &c., at different Seasons of the Year; and an Appendix on the Mineral Springs of the Pyrenees, Vichy, and Aix les Bains. Post 8vo. cloth, 8s. 6d.

C. REMIGIUS FRESENIUS.

ELEMENTARY INSTRUCTION IN CHEMICAL ANALYSIS, AS PRACTISED IN THE LABORATORY OF GIESSEN. Edited by LLOYD BULLOCK, late Student at Giessen.

QUALITATIVE; Fourth Edition.   8vo. cloth, 9s.
QUANTITATIVE. Second Edition.   8vo. cloth, 15s.

MR. FOWNES, PH.D., F.R.S.

I.

A MANUAL OF CHEMISTRY; with numerous Illustrations on Wood.
Sixth Edition. Fcap. 8vo. cloth, 12s. 6d.
Edited by H. BENCE JONES, M.D., F.R.S., and A. W. HOFMANN, PH.D., F.R.S.

II.

CHEMISTRY, AS EXEMPLIFYING THE WISDOM AND BENEFICENCE OF GOD. Second Edition. Fcap. 8vo. cloth, 4s. 6d.

III.

INTRODUCTION TO QUALITATIVE ANALYSIS. Post 8vo. cloth, 2s.

IV.

CHEMICAL TABLES. Folio, price 2s. 6d.

DR. FULLER.

ON RHEUMATISM, RHEUMATIC GOUT, AND SCIATICA: their Pathology, Symptoms, and Treatment. Second Edition. 8vo. cloth, 12s. 6d.

DR. GAIRDNER.

ON GOUT; its History, its Causes, and its Cure. Third Edition. Post 8vo. cloth, 8s. 6d.

MR. GALLOWAY.

I.

THE FIRST STEP IN CHEMISTRY. Second Edition. Fcap. 8vo. cloth, 5s.

II.

A MANUAL OF QUALITATIVE ANALYSIS. Second Edition. Post 8vo. cloth, 4s. 6d.

III.

CHEMICAL DIAGRAMS. On Four large Sheets, for School and Lecture Rooms. 5s. 6d. the Set.

MR. ROBERT GARNER, F.L.S.

EUTHERAPEIA; or, AN EXAMINATION OF THE PRINCIPLES OF MEDICAL SCIENCE, including Researches on the Nervous System. Illustrated with 9 Engravings on Copper, and Engravings on Wood. 8vo. cloth, 8s.

DR. GARRETT.

ON EAST AND NORTH-EAST WINDS; the Nature, Treatment, and Prevention of their Suffocating Effects. Fcap. 8vo. cloth, 4s. 6d.

MR. GAY, F.R.C.S.E.

I.

FEMORAL RUPTURE: ITS ANATOMY, PATHOLOGY, AND SURGERY. With a New Mode of Operating. 4to., Plates, 10s. 6d.

II.

A MEMOIR ON INDOLENT ULCERS. Post 8vo. cloth, 3s. 6d.

DR. GRANVILLE, F.R.S.

ON SUDDEN DEATH. Post 8vo., 2s. 6d.

MR. GRAY, M.R.C.S.

PRESERVATION OF THE TEETH indispensable to Comfort and Appearance, Health, and Longevity. 18mo. cloth, 3s.

MR. GRIFFITHS.

CHEMISTRY OF THE FOUR SEASONS — Spring, Summer, Autumn, Winter. Illustrated with Engravings on Wood. Second Edition. Foolscap 8vo. cloth, 7s. 6d.

DR. GULLY.

I.

THE WATER CURE IN CHRONIC DISEASE: an Exposition of the Causes, Progress, and Terminations of various Chronic Diseases of the Viscera, Nervous System, and Limbs, and of their Treatment by Water and other Hygienic Means. Fifth Edition. Foolscap 8vo. sewed, 2s. 6d.

II.

THE SIMPLE TREATMENT OF DISEASE; deduced from the Methods of Expectancy and Revulsion. 18mo. cloth, 4s.

DR. GUY.

HOOPER'S PHYSICIAN'S VADE-MECUM; OR, MANUAL OF THE PRINCIPLES AND PRACTICE OF PHYSIC. New Edition, considerably enlarged, and rewritten. Foolscap 8vo. cloth, 12s. 6d.

GUY'S HOSPITAL REPORTS. Third Series. Vols. I. to III., 8vo., 7s. 6d. each.

DR. HABERSHON.

OBSERVATIONS ON DISEASES OF THE ALIMENTARY CANAL, ŒSOPHAGUS, STOMACH, CÆCUM, and INTESTINES. 8vo. cloth, 10s. 6d.

DR. MARSHALL HALL, F.R.S.

I.

PRONE AND POSTURAL RESPIRATION IN DROWNING AND OTHER FORMS OF APNŒA OR SUSPENDED RESPIRATION. Post 8vo. cloth. 5s.

II.

PRACTICAL OBSERVATIONS AND SUGGESTIONS IN MEDI-CINE. Post 8vo. cloth, 8s. 6d.

DITTO. Second Series. Post 8vo. cloth, 8s. 6d.

DR. C. RADCLYFFE HALL.

TORQUAY IN ITS MEDICAL ASPECT AS A RESORT FOR PULMONARY INVALIDS. Post 8vo. cloth, 5s.

MR. HARDWICH.

A MANUAL OF PHOTOGRAPHIC CHEMISTRY. Fourth Edition. Foolscap 8vo. cloth, 6s. 6d.

MR. HARE, M.R.C.S.

PRACTICAL OBSERVATIONS ON THE PREVENTION, CAUSES, AND TREATMENT OF CURVATURES OF THE SPINE; with Engravings. Third Edition. 8vo. cloth, 6s.

MR. HARRISON, F.R.C.S.

THE PATHOLOGY AND TREATMENT OF STRICTURE OF THE URETHRA. 8vo. cloth, 7s. 6d.

MR. JAMES B. HARRISON, F.R.C.S.

ON THE CONTAMINATION OF WATER BY THE POISON OF LEAD, and its Effects on the Human Body. Foolscap 8vo. cloth, 3s. 6d.

DR. HARTWIG.

I.

ON SEA BATHING AND SEA AIR. Fcap. 8vo., 2s. 6d.

II.

ON THE PHYSICAL EDUCATION OF CHILDREN. Fcap. 8vo., 2s. 6d.

DR. A. H. HASSALL.

THE MICROSCOPIC ANATOMY OF THE HUMAN BODY, IN HEALTH AND DISEASE. Illustrated with Several Hundred Drawings in Colour. Two vols. 8vo. cloth, £1. 10s.

MR. ALFRED HAVILAND, M.R.C.S.

CLIMATE, WEATHER, AND DISEASE; being a Sketch of the Opinions of the most celebrated Ancient and Modern Writers with regard to the Influence of Climate and Weather in producing Disease. With Four coloured Engravings. 8vo. cloth, 7s.

DR. HEADLAND.

ON THE ACTION OF MEDICINES IN THE SYSTEM. Being the Prize Essay to which the Medical Society of London awarded the Fothergillian Gold Medal for 1852. Second Edition. 8vo. cloth, 10s.

MR. HIGGINBOTTOM, F.R.S., F.R.C.S.

I.

AN ESSAY ON THE USE OF THE NITRATE OF SILVER IN THE CURE OF INFLAMMATION, WOUNDS, AND ULCERS. Second Edition. Price 5s.

II.

ADDITIONAL OBSERVATIONS ON THE NITRATE OF SILVER; with full Directions for its Use as a Therapeutic Agent. 8vo., 2s. 6d.

MR. JOHN HILTON, F.R.S.

ON THE DEVELOPMENT AND DESIGN OF CERTAIN PORTIONS OF THE CRANIUM. Illustrated with Plates in Lithography. 8vo. cloth, 6s.

DR. HINDS.

THE HARMONIES OF PHYSICAL SCIENCE IN RELATION TO THE HIGHER SENTIMENTS; with Observations on Medical Studies, and on the Moral and Scientific Relations of Medical Life. Post 8vo., cloth, 5s.

DR. DECIMUS HODGSON.

THE PROSTATE GLAND, AND ITS ENLARGEMENT IN OLD AGE. With 12 Plates. Royal 8vo., cloth, 6s.

MR. LUTHER HOLDEN, F.R.C.S.

HUMAN OSTEOLOGY : with Plates, showing the Attachments of the Muscles. Second Edition. 8vo. cloth, 16s.

DR. G. CALVERT HOLLAND.

THE CONSTITUTION OF THE ANIMAL CREATION, expressed in Structural Appendages, as Hair, Horns, Tusks, and Fat. 8vo. cloth, 10s. 6d.

MR. C. HOLTHOUSE.

I.

ON SQUINTING, PARALYTIC AFFECTIONS OF THE EYE, and CERTAIN FORMS OF IMPAIRED VISION. Fcap. 8vo. cloth, 4s. 6d.

II.

LECTURES ON STRABISMUS, delivered at the Westminster Hospital. 8vo. cloth, 4s.

DR. W. CHARLES HOOD.

SUGGESTIONS FOR THE FUTURE PROVISION OF CRIMI-
NAL LUNATICS.   8vo. cloth, 5s. 6d.

MR. P. HOOD.

THE SUCCESSFUL TREATMENT OF SCARLET FEVER;
also, OBSERVATIONS ON THE PATHOLOGY AND TREATMENT OF
CROWING INSPIRATIONS OF INFANTS.   Post 8vo. cloth, 5s.

DR. HOOPER.

THE MEDICAL DICTIONARY; containing an Explanation of the
Terms used in Medicine and the Collateral Sciences.   Eighth Edition.   Edited by
KLEIN GRANT, M.D.   8vo. cloth, 30s.

MR. JOHN HORSLEY.

A CATECHISM OF CHEMICAL PHILOSOPHY; being a Familiar
Exposition of the Principles of Chemistry and Physics.   With Engravings on Wood.
Designed for the Use of Schools and Private Teachers.   Post 8vo. cloth, 6s. 6d.

DR. HUFELAND.

THE ART OF PROLONGING LIFE.   A New Edition.   Edited
by ERASMUS WILSON, F.R.S.   Foolscap 8vo., 2s. 6d.

DR. HENRY HUNT.

ON HEARTBURN AND INDIGESTION.   8vo. cloth, 5s.

MR. T. HUNT.

DISEASES OF THE SKIN: a Guide for their Treatment and Prevention.   Second Edition.   Fcap. 8vo., 2s. 6d.

DR. INMAN.

THE PHENOMENA OF SPINAL IRRITATION AND OTHER
FUNCTIONAL DISEASES OF THE NERVOUS SYSTEM EXPLAINED,
and a Rational Plan of Treatment deduced.   With Plates.   8vo. cloth, 6s.

DR. ARTHUR JACOB, F.R.C.S.

A TREATISE ON THE INFLAMMATIONS OF THE EYE-BALL.
Foolscap 8vo. cloth, 5s.

DR. JAMES JAGO, A.B., CANTAB.; M.B., OXON.

OCULAR SPECTRES AND STRUCTURES AS MUTUAL EXPO-
NENTS.   Illustrated with Engravings on Wood.   8vo. cloth, 5s.

DR. HANDFIELD JONES, F.R.S.

PATHOLOGICAL AND CLINICAL OBSERVATIONS RESPECT-
ING MORBID CONDITIONS OF THE STOMACH.   Coloured Plates, 8vo. cloth, 9s.

DR. HANDFIELD JONES, F.R.S., & DR. EDWARD H. SIEVEKING.

A MANUAL OF PATHOLOGICAL ANATOMY. Illustrated with numerous Engravings on Wood. Foolscap 8vo. cloth, 12s. 6d.

MR. WHARTON JONES, F.R.S.

I.

A MANUAL OF THE PRINCIPLES AND PRACTICE OF OPHTHALMIC MEDICINE AND SURGERY; illustrated with Engravings, plain and coloured. Second Edition. Foolscap 8vo. cloth, 12s. 6d.

II.

THE WISDOM AND BENEFICENCE OF THE ALMIGHTY, AS DISPLAYED IN THE SENSE OF VISION; being the Actonian Prize Essay for 1851. With Illustrations on Steel and Wood. Foolscap 8vo. cloth, 4s. 6d.

III.

DEFECTS OF SIGHT: their Nature, Causes, Prevention, and General Management. Fcap. 8vo. 2s. 6d.

IV.

A CATECHISM OF THE MEDICINE AND SURGERY OF THE EYE AND EAR. For the Clinical Use of Hospital Students. Fcap. 8vo. 2s. 6d.

DR. BENCE JONES, F.R.S.

I.

MULDER ON WINE. Foolscap 8vo. cloth, 6s.

II.

ON ANIMAL CHEMISTRY, in its relation to STOMACH and RENAL DISEASES. 8vo. cloth, 6s.

MR. JUDD.

A PRACTICAL TREATISE ON URETHRITIS AND SYPHI-LIS: including Observations on the Power of the Menstruous Fluid, and of the Discharge from Leucorrhœa and Sores to produce Urethritis: with a variety of Examples, Experiments, Remedies, and Cures. 8vo. cloth, £1. 5s.

MR. KNAGGS.

UNSOUNDNESS OF MIND CONSIDERED IN RELATION TO THE QUESTION OF RESPONSIBILITY IN CRIMINAL CASES. 8vo. cloth, 4s. 6d.

DR. LAENNEC.

A MANUAL OF AUSCULTATION AND PERCUSSION. Translated and Edited by J. B. SHARPE, M.R.C.S. 3s.

DR. HUNTER LANE, F.L.S.

A COMPENDIUM OF MATERIA MEDICA AND PHARMACY; adapted to the London Pharmacopœia, 1851, embodying all the new French, American, and Indian Medicines, and also comprising a Summary of Practical Toxicology. Second Edition. 24mo. cloth, 5s. 6d.

DR. LANE, M.A.

HYDROPATHY; OR, THE NATURAL SYSTEM OF MEDICAL
TREATMENT. An Explanatory Essay. Post 8vo. cloth, 3s. 6d.

MR. LAURENCE, M.B., F.R.C.S.

THE DIAGNOSIS OF SURGICAL CANCER. The Liston Prize
Essay for 1854. Plates, 8vo. cloth, 4s. 6d.

MR. LAWRENCE, F.R.S.

A TREATISE ON RUPTURES. The Fifth Edition, considerably
enlarged. 8vo. cloth, 16s.

DR. EDWIN LEE.

I.

THE EFFECT OF CLIMATE ON TUBERCULOUS DISEASE,
with Notices of the chief Foreign Places of Winter Resort. Small 8vo. cloth, 6s.

II.

THE WATERING PLACES OF ENGLAND, CONSIDERED
with Reference to their Medical Topography. Third Edition. Foolscap 8vo. cloth,
5s. 6d.

III.

THE BATHS OF GERMANY, FRANCE, & SWITZERLAND.
Third Edition. Post 8vo. cloth, 8s. 6d.

IV.

THE BATHS OF RHENISH GERMANY. Post 8vo. cloth, 4s.

MR. HENRY LEE, F.R.C.S.

PATHOLOGICAL AND SURGICAL OBSERVATIONS; including
an Essay on the Surgical Treatment of Hemorrhoidal Tumors. 8vo. cloth, 7s. 6d.

DR. ROBERT LEE, F.R.S.

I.

CLINICAL REPORTS OF OVARIAN AND UTERINE DIS-
EASES, with Commentaries. Foolscap 8vo. cloth, 6s. 6d.

II.

CLINICAL MIDWIFERY: comprising the Histories of 545 Cases of
Difficult, Preternatural, and Complicated Labour, with Commentaries. Second Edition.
Foolscap 8vo. cloth, 5s.

III.

PRACTICAL OBSERVATIONS ON DISEASES OF THE
UTERUS. With coloured Plates. Two Parts. Imperial 4to., 7s. 6d. each Part.

MR. LISTON, F.R.S.

PRACTICAL SURGERY. Fourth Edition. 8vo. cloth, 22s.

MR. H. W. LOBB, L.S.A., M.R.C.S.E.

ON SOME OF THE MORE OBSCURE FORMS OF NERVOUS AFFECTIONS, THEIR PATHOLOGY AND TREATMENT. With an Introduction on the Physiology of Digestion and Assimilation, and the Generation and Distribution of Nerve Force. Based upon Original Microscopical Observations. With Engravings. 8vo. cloth, 10s. 6d.

LONDON MEDICAL SOCIETY OF OBSERVATION.

WHAT TO OBSERVE AT THE BED-SIDE, AND AFTER DEATH. Published by Authority. Second Edition. Foolscap 8vo. cloth, 4s. 6d.

M. LUGOL.

ON SCROFULOUS DISEASES. Translated from the French, with Additions by W. H. RANKING, M.D., Physician to the Suffolk General Hospital. 8vo. cloth, 10s. 6d.

MR. JOSEPH MACLISE, F.R.C.S.

I.

SURGICAL ANATOMY. A Series of Dissections, illustrating the Principal Regions of the Human Body.

The Second Edition, complete in XIII. Fasciculi. Imperial folio, 5s. each; bound in cloth, £3. 12s.; or bound in morocco, £4. 4s.

II.

ON DISLOCATIONS AND FRACTURES. This Work will be Uniform with the Author's "Surgical Anatomy;" each Fasciculus will contain Four beautifully executed Lithographic Drawings, and be completed in Nine Numbers. Fasciculus I., imperial folio, 5s.

DR. MAYNE.

AN EXPOSITORY LEXICON OF THE TERMS, ANCIENT AND MODERN, IN MEDICAL AND GENERAL SCIENCE, including a complete MEDICAL AND MEDICO-LEGAL VOCABULARY, and presenting the correct Pronunciation, Derivation, Definition, and Explanation of the Names, Analogues, Synonymes, and Phrases (in English, Latin, Greek, French, and German,) employed in Science and connected with Medicine. Parts I. to VI., price 5s. each.

DR. WM. H. MADDEN.

THOUGHTS ON PULMONARY CONSUMPTION; with an Appendix on the Climate of Torquay. Post 8vo. cloth, 5s.

DR. MARCET.

ON THE COMPOSITION OF FOOD, AND HOW IT IS ADULTERATED; with Practical Directions for its Analysis. 8vo. cloth, 6s. 6d.

DR. MARTIN.

THE UNDERCLIFF, ISLE OF WIGHT: its Climate, History, and Natural Productions. Post 8vo. cloth, 10s. 6d.

DR. MARKHAM.

I.

DISEASES OF THE HEART: THEIR PATHOLOGY, DIAGNOSIS, AND TREATMENT. Post. 8vo. cloth, 6s.

II.

SKODA ON AUSCULTATION AND PERCUSSION. Post 8vo. cloth, 6s.

MR. J. RANALD MARTIN, F.R.S.

THE INFLUENCE OF TROPICAL CLIMATES ON EUROPEAN CONSTITUTIONS. Originally by the late JAMES JOHNSON, M.D., and now entirely rewritten; including Practical Observations on the Diseases of European Invalids on their Return from Tropical Climates. Seventh Edition. 8vo. cloth, 16s.

DR. MASSY.

ON THE EXAMINATION OF RECRUITS; intended for the Use of Young Medical Officers on Entering the Army. 8vo. cloth, 5s.

DR. MILLINGEN.

ON THE TREATMENT AND MANAGEMENT OF THE INSANE; with Considerations on Public and Private Lunatic Asylums. 18mo. cloth, 4s. 6d.

MR. JOHN L. MILTON, M.R.C.S.

PRACTICAL OBSERVATIONS ON A NEW WAY OF TREATING GONORRHŒA. With some Remarks on the Cure of Inveterate Cases. 8vo. cloth, 5s.

DR. MONRO.

I.

REMARKS ON INSANITY: its Nature and Treatment. 8vo. cloth, 6s.

II.

REFORM IN PRIVATE LUNATIC ASYLUMS. 8vo. cloth, 4s.

DR. NOBLE.

ELEMENTS OF PSYCHOLOGICAL MEDICINE: AN INTRODUCTION TO THE PRACTICAL STUDY OF INSANITY. Second Edition. 8vo. cloth, 10s.

MR. J. NOTTINGHAM, F.R.C.S.

I.

DISEASES OF THE EAR. Illustrated by Clinical Observations. 8vo. cloth, 12s.

II.

PRACTICAL OBSERVATIONS ON CONICAL CORNEA, AND on the Short Sight, and other Defects of Vision connected with it. 8vo. cloth, 6s.

MR. NOURSE, M.R.C.S.

TABLES FOR STUDENTS. Price One Shilling.

1. Divisions and Classes of the Animal Kingdom.
2. Classes and Orders of the Vertebrate Sub-kingdom.
3. Classes of the Vegetable Kingdom, according to the Natural and Artificial Systems.
4. Table of the Elements, with their Chemical Equivalents and Symbols.

MR. NUNNELEY.

A TREATISE ON THE NATURE, CAUSES, AND TREATMENT
OF ERYSIPELAS. 8vo. cloth, 10s. 6d.

𝔒𝔯𝔣𝔬𝔯𝔡 𝔈𝔡𝔦𝔱𝔦𝔬𝔫𝔰.—Edited by DR. GREENHILL.

I. ADDRESS TO A MEDICAL STUDENT. Second Edition, 18mo. cloth, 2s. 6d.

II. PRAYERS FOR THE USE OF THE MEDICAL PROFESSION. Second Edition, cloth, 1s. 6d.

III. LIFE OF SIR JAMES STONHOUSE, BART., M.D. Cloth, 4s. 6d.

IV. ANECDOTA SYDENHAMIANA. Second Edition, 18mo. 2s.

V. LIFE OF THOMAS HARRISON BURDER, M.D. 18mo. cloth, 4s.

VI. BURDER'S LETTERS FROM A SENIOR TO A JUNIOR PHYSICIAN, ON PROMOTING THE RELIGIOUS WELFARE OF HIS PATIENTS. 18mo. sewed, 6d.

VII. LIFE OF GEORGE CHEYNE, M.D. 18mo. sewed, 2s. 6d.

VIII. HUFELAND ON THE RELATIONS OF THE PHYSICIAN TO THE SICK, TO THE PUBLIC, AND TO HIS COLLEAGUES. 18mo. sewed, 9d.

IX. GISBORNE ON THE DUTIES OF PHYSICIANS. 18mo. sewed, 1s.

X. LIFE OF CHARLES BRANDON TRYE. 18mo. sewed, 1s.

XI. PERCIVAL'S MEDICAL ETHICS. Third Edition, 18mo. cloth, 3s.

XII. CODE OF ETHICS OF THE AMERICAN MEDICAL ASSOCIATION. 8d.

XIII. WARE ON THE DUTIES AND QUALIFICATIONS OF PHYSICIANS. 8d.

XIV. MAURICE ON THE RESPONSIBILITIES OF MEDICAL STUDENTS. 9d.

XV. FRASER'S QUERIES IN MEDICAL ETHICS. 9d.

DR. ODLING.

A COURSE OF PRACTICAL CHEMISTRY, FOR THE USE
OF MEDICAL STUDENTS. Arranged with express reference to the Three Months' Summer Course. Post 8vo. cloth, 4s. 6d.

MR. PAGET.

A DESCRIPTIVE CATALOGUE OF THE ANATOMICAL
MUSEUM OF ST. BARTHOLOMEW'S HOSPITAL. VOL. I. Morbid Anatomy. 8vo. cloth, 5s.

DITTO. Vol. II. Natural and Congenitally Malformed Structures, and Lists of the Models, Casts, Drawings, and Diagrams. 5s.

MR. LANGSTON PARKER.

THE MODERN TREATMENT OF SYPHILITIC DISEASES,

both Primary and Secondary; comprising the Treatment of Constitutional and Confirmed Syphilis, by a safe and successful Method. Third Edition, 8vo. cloth, 10s.

MR. JAMES PART, F.R.C.S.

THE MEDICAL AND SURGICAL POCKET CASE BOOK,

for the Registration of important Cases in Private Practice, and to assist the Student of Hospital Practice. Second Edition. 3s. 6d.

DR. THOMAS B. PEACOCK, M.D.

ON THE INFLUENZA, OR EPIDEMIC CATARRHAL FEVER

OF 1847-8. 8vo. cloth, 5s. 6d.

DR. PEREIRA, F.R.S.

SELECTA E PRÆSCRIPTIS. Twelfth Edition. 24mo. cloth, 5s.

MR. PETTIGREW, F.R.S.

ON SUPERSTITIONS connected with the History and Practice of

Medicine and Surgery. 8vo. cloth, 7s.

MR. PIRRIE, F.R.S.E.

THE PRINCIPLES AND PRACTICE OF SURGERY. With

numerous Engravings on Wood. 8vo. cloth, 21s.

PHARMACOPŒIA COLLEGII REGALIS MEDICORUM LON-

DINENSIS. 8vo. cloth, 9s.; or 24mo. 5s.

IMPRIMATUR.

Hic liber, cui titulus, PHARMACOPŒIA COLLEGII REGALIS MEDICORUM LONDINENSIS. Datum ex Ædibus Collegii in comitiis censoriis, Novembris Mensis 14to 1850.

JOHANNES AYRTON PARIS. *Præses.*

PROFESSORS PLATTNER & MUSPRATT.

THE USE OF THE BLOWPIPE IN THE EXAMINATION OF

MINERALS, ORES, AND OTHER METALLIC COMBINATIONS. Illustrated by numerous Engravings on Wood. Third Edition. 8vo. cloth, 10s. 6d.

THE PRESCRIBER'S PHARMACOPŒIA; containing all the Medi-

cines in the London Pharmacopœia, arranged in Classes according to their Action, with their Composition and Doses. By a Practising Physician. Fourth Edition. 32mo. cloth, 2s. 6d.; roan tuck (for the pocket), 3s. 6d.

DR. JOHN ROWLISON PRETTY.

AIDS DURING LABOUR, including the Administration of Chloroform, the Management of Placenta and Post-partum Hæmorrhage. Fcap. 8vo. cloth, 4s. 6d.

SIR WM. PYM, K.C.H.

OBSERVATIONS UPON YELLOW FEVER, with a Review of "A Report upon the Diseases of the African Coast, by Sir WM. BURNETT and Dr. BRYSON," proving its highly Contagious Powers. Post 8vo. 6s.

DR. RADCLIFFE.

EPILEPSY, AND OTHER AFFECTIONS OF THE NERVOUS SYSTEM which are marked by Tremor, Convulsion, or Spasm: their Pathology and Treatment. 8vo. cloth, 5s.

DR. F. H. RAMSBOTHAM.

THE PRINCIPLES AND PRACTICE OF OBSTETRIC MEDI-CINE AND SURGERY. Illustrated with One Hundred and Twenty Plates on Steel and Wood; forming one thick handsome volume. Fourth Edition. 8vo. cloth, 22s.

DR. RAMSBOTHAM.

PRACTICAL OBSERVATIONS ON MIDWIFERY, with a Selection of Cases. Second Edition. 8vo. cloth, 12s.

DR. DU BOIS REYMOND.

ANIMAL ELECTRICITY; Edited by H. BENCE JONES, M.D., F.R.S. With Fifty Engravings on Wood. Foolscap 8vo. cloth, 6s.

DR. REYNOLDS.

THE DIAGNOSIS OF DISEASES OF THE BRAIN, SPINAL CORD, AND THEIR APPENDAGES. 8vo. cloth, 8s.

DR. B. W. RICHARDSON.
I.

ON THE CAUSE OF THE COAGULATION OF THE BLOOD. Being the ASTLEY COOPER PRIZE ESSAY for 1856. With a Practical Appendix. 8vo. cloth.

II.

THE HYGIENIC TREATMENT OF PULMONARY CONSUMP-TION. 8vo. cloth, 5s. 6d.

DR. W. H. ROBERTSON.
I.

THE NATURE AND TREATMENT OF GOUT. 8vo. cloth, 10s. 6d.

II.

A TREATISE ON DIET AND REGIMEN. Fourth Edition. 2 vols. post 8vo. cloth, 12s.

MR. ROBERTON.

ON THE PHYSIOLOGY AND DISEASES OF WOMEN, AND
ON PRACTICAL MIDWIFERY.   8vo. cloth, 12s.

DR. ROTH.

ON MOVEMENTS. An Exposition of their Principles and Practice, for
the Correction of the Tendencies to Disease in Infancy, Childhood, and Youth, and for
the Cure of many Morbid Affections in Adults.   Illustrated with numerous Engravings
on Wood.   8vo. cloth, 10s.

DR. ROWE, F.S.A.

I.

ON SOME OF THE MORE IMPORTANT DISEASES OF
WOMEN and CHILDREN.   Second Edition.   Fcap. 8vo. cloth, 4s. 6d.

II.

NERVOUS DISEASES, LIVER AND STOMACH COM-
PLAINTS, LOW SPIRITS, INDIGESTION, GOUT, ASTHMA, AND DIS-
ORDERS PRODUCED BY TROPICAL CLIMATES.   With Cases.   Fifteenth
Edition.   Fcap. 8vo. 2s. 6d.

DR. ROYLE, F.R.S.

A MANUAL OF MATERIA MEDICA AND THERAPEUTICS.
With numerous Engravings on Wood.   Third Edition.   Fcap. 8vo. cloth, 12s. 6d.

MR. RUMSEY, F.R.C.S.

ESSAYS ON STATE MEDICINE. 8vo. cloth, 10s. 6d.

MR. SAVORY.

A COMPENDIUM OF DOMESTIC MEDICINE, AND COMPA-
NION TO THE MEDICINE CHEST; comprising Plain Directions for the Employment of Medicines, with their Properties and Doses, and Brief Descriptions of the
Symptoms and Treatment of Diseases, and of the Disorders incidental to Infants and
Children, with a Selection of the most efficacious Prescriptions.   Intended as a Source
of Easy Reference for Clergymen, and for Families residing at a Distance from Profes-
sional Assistance.   Fifth Edition.   12mo. cloth, 5s.

DR. SCHACHT.

THE MICROSCOPE, AND ITS APPLICATION TO VEGETABLE
ANATOMY AND PHYSIOLOGY.   Edited by Frederick Currey, M.A.   Fcap.
8vo. cloth, 6s.

DR. SEMPLE.

ON COUGH : its Causes, Varieties, and Treatment. With some practical
Remarks on the Use of the Stethoscope as an aid to Diagnosis.   Post 8vo. cloth, 4s. 6d.

MR. SHAW, M.R.C.S.

THE MEDICAL REMEMBRANCER ; OR, BOOK OF EMER-
GENCIES : in which are concisely pointed out the Immediate Remedies to be adopted
in the First Moments of Danger from Poisoning, Drowning, Apoplexy, Burns, and other
Accidents; with the Tests for the Principal Poisons, and other useful Information.
Fourth Edition. Edited, with Additions, by JONATHAN HUTCHINSON, M.R.C.S. 32mo.
cloth, 2s. 6d.

DR. SIBSON, F.R.S.

MEDICAL ANATOMY. With coloured Plates. Imperial folio. Fasciculi I. to V. 5s. each.

DR. E. H. SIEVEKING.

ON EPILEPSY AND EPILEPTIFORM SEIZURES : their
Causes, Pathology, and Treatment. Post 8vo. cloth, 7s. 6d.

MR. SKEY, F.R.S.

OPERATIVE SURGERY : with Illustrations engraved on Wood. 8vo.
cloth, 12s. 6d.

DR. SMELLIE.

OBSTETRIC PLATES : being a Selection from the more Important and
Practical Illustrations contained in the Original Work. With Anatomical and Practical
Directions. 8vo. cloth, 5s.

MR. HENRY SMITH, F.R.C.S.

ON STRICTURE OF THE URETHRA. 8vo. cloth, 7s. 6d.

DR. W. TYLER SMITH.

I.

THE PATHOLOGY AND TREATMENT OF LEUCORRHŒA.
With Engravings on Wood. 8vo. cloth, 7s.

II.

THE PERIODOSCOPE, a new Instrument for determining the Date of
Labour, and other Obstetric Calculations, with an Explanation of its Uses, and an Essay
on the Periodic Phenomena attending Pregnancy and Parturition. 8vo. cloth, 4s.

DR. SNOW.

ON THE MODE OF COMMUNICATION OF CHOLERA.
Second Edition, much Enlarged, and Illustrated with Maps. 8vo. cloth, 7s.

DR. STANHOPE TEMPLEMAN SPEER.

PATHOLOGICAL CHEMISTRY, IN ITS APPLICATION TO
THE PRACTICE OF MEDICINE. Translated from the French of MM. BECQUEREL
and RODIER. 8vo. cloth, 12s.

DR. SPURGIN.

LECTURES ON MATERIA MEDICA, AND ITS RELATIONS
TO THE ANIMAL ECONOMY. Delivered before the Royal College of Physicians.
8vo. cloth, 5s. 6d.

MR. SQUIRE.

THE PHARMACOPŒIA, (LONDON, EDINBURGH, AND
DUBLIN,) arranged in a convenient TABULAR FORM, both to suit the Prescriber for
comparison, and the Dispenser for compounding the formulæ; with Notes, Tests, and
Tables. 8vo. cloth, 12s.

DR. SWAYNE.

OBSTETRIC APHORISMS FOR THE USE OF STUDENTS
COMMENCING MIDWIFERY PRACTICE. With Engravings on Wood. Fcap.
8vo. cloth, 3s. 6d.

DR. STEGGALL.
STUDENTS' BOOKS FOR EXAMINATION.

I.

A MEDICAL MANUAL FOR APOTHECARIES' HALL AND OTHER MEDICAL
BOARDS. Eleventh Edition. 12mo. cloth, 10s.

II.

A MANUAL FOR THE COLLEGE OF SURGEONS; intended for the Use
of Candidates for Examination and Practitioners. Second Edition. 12mo. cloth, 10s.

III.

GREGORY'S CONSPECTUS MEDICINÆ THEORETICÆ. The First Part, con-
taining the Original Text, with an Ordo Verborum, and Literal Translation. 12mo.
cloth, 10s.

IV.

THE FIRST FOUR BOOKS OF CELSUS; containing the Text, Ordo Verb-
orum, and Translation. Second Edition. 12mo. cloth, 8s.

V.

A TEXT-BOOK OF MATERIA-MEDICA AND THERAPEUTICS. 12mo. cloth, 7s.

VI.

FIRST LINES FOR CHEMISTS AND DRUGGISTS PREPARING FOR EX-
AMINATION AT THE PHARMACEUTICAL SOCIETY. Second Edition.
18mo. cloth, 3s. 6d.

MR. STOWE, M.R.C.S.

A TOXICOLOGICAL CHART, exhibiting at one view the Symptoms,
Treatment, and Mode of Detecting the various Poisons, Mineral, Vegetable, and Animal.
To which are added, concise Directions for the Treatment of Suspended Animation.
Eleventh Edition. On Sheet, 2s.; mounted on Roller, 5s.

MR. TAMPLIN, F.R.C.S.E.

LATERAL CURVATURE OF THE SPINE: its Causes, Nature, and Treatment. 8vo. cloth, 4s.

DR. ALFRED S. TAYLOR, F.R.S.

I.

A MANUAL OF MEDICAL JURISPRUDENCE. Fifth Edition. Fcap. 8vo. cloth, 12s. 6d.

II.

ON POISONS, in relation to MEDICAL JURISPRUDENCE AND MEDICINE. Fcap. 8vo. cloth, 12s. 6d.

DR. THEOPHILUS THOMPSON, F.R.S.

I.

CLINICAL LECTURES ON PULMONARY CONSUMPTION. With Plates. 8vo. cloth, 7s. 6d.

II.

LETTSOMIAN LECTURES ON PULMONARY CONSUMPTION; with Remarks on Microscopical Indications, and on Cocoa-nut Oil. Post 8vo., 2s. 6d.

DR. THOMAS.

THE MODERN PRACTICE OF PHYSIC; exhibiting the Symptoms, Causes, Morbid Appearances, and Treatment of the Diseases of all Climates. Eleventh Edition. Revised by ALGERNON FRAMPTON, M.D. 2 vols. 8vo. cloth, 28s.

HENRY THOMPSON, M.B. LOND., F.R.C.S.

STRICTURE OF THE URETHRA; its Pathology and Treatment. The last Jacksonian Treatise of the Royal College of Surgeons. With Plates. 8vo. cloth, 10s.

DR. TILT.

I.

ON DISEASES OF WOMEN AND OVARIAN INFLAM-MATION IN RELATION TO MORBID MENSTRUATION, STERILITY, PELVIC TUMOURS, AND AFFECTIONS OF THE WOMB. Second Edition. 8vo. cloth, 9s.

II.

THE CHANGE OF LIFE IN HEALTH AND DISEASE: a Practical Treatise on the Nervous and other Affections incidental to Women at the Decline of Life. Second Edition. 8vo. cloth, 6s.

DR. ROBERT B. TODD, F.R.S.

I.

CLINICAL LECTURES ON PARALYSIS, DISEASES OF THE
BRAIN, and other AFFECTIONS of the NERVOUS SYSTEM. Second Edition.
Foolscap 8vo. cloth, 6s.

II.

CLINICAL LECTURES ON CERTAIN DISEASES OF THE
URINARY ORGANS, AND ON DROPSIES. Fcap. 8vo. cloth, 6s.

MR. JOSEPH TOYNBEE, F.R.S.

A DESCRIPTIVE CATALOGUE OF PREPARATIONS ILLUS-
TRATIVE OF THE DISEASES OF THE EAR, IN HIS MUSEUM. 8vo.
cloth, 5s.

MR. SAMUEL TUKE.

DR. JACOBI ON THE CONSTRUCTION AND MANAGEMENT
OF HOSPITALS FOR THE INSANE. Translated from the German. With In-
troductory Observations by the Editor. With Plates. 8vo. cloth, 9s.

DR. TURNBULL.

A PRACTICAL TREATISE ON DISORDERS OF THE STOMACH
with FERMENTATION; and on the Causes and Treatment of Indigestion, &c. 8vo.
cloth, 6s.

DR. UNDERWOOD.

TREATISE ON THE DISEASES OF CHILDREN. Tenth Edition,
with Additions and Corrections by HENRY DAVIES, M.D. 8vo. cloth, 15s.

VESTIGES OF THE NATURAL HISTORY OF CREATION.
Tenth Edition. Illustrated with 100 Engravings on Wood. 8vo. cloth, 12s. 6d.

BY THE SAME AUTHOR.

EXPLANATIONS: A SEQUEL TO "VESTIGES."
Second Edition. Post 8vo. cloth, 5s.

DR. UNGER.

BOTANICAL LETTERS. Translated by Dr. B. PAUL. Numerous
Woodcuts. Post 8vo., 5s.

DR. VAN OVEN.

ON THE DECLINE OF LIFE IN HEALTH AND DISEASE;
being an Attempt to Investigate the Causes of LONGEVITY, and the Best Means of Attaining a Healthful Old Age. 8vo. cloth, 10s. 6d.

MR. WADE, F.R.C.S.

STRICTURE OF THE URETHRA; its Complications and Effects.
With Practical Observations on its Causes, Symptoms, and Treatment; and on a Safe and Efficient Mode of Treating its more Intractable Forms. 8vo. cloth, 5s.

MR. HAYNES WALTON, F.R.C.S.

OPERATIVE OPHTHALMIC SURGERY. With Engravings on
Wood. 8vo. cloth, 18s.

DR. WARDROP.

ON DISEASES OF THE HEART. 8vo. cloth, 12s.

DR. EBEN. WATSON, A.M.

ON THE TOPICAL MEDICATION OF THE LARYNX IN
CERTAIN DISEASES OF THE RESPIRATORY AND VOCAL ORGANS. 8vo. cloth, 5s.

DR. WEBER.

A CLINICAL HAND-BOOK OF AUSCULTATION AND PER-
CUSSION. Translated by JOHN COCKLE, M.D. 5s.

DR. WEGG.

OBSERVATIONS RELATING TO THE SCIENCE AND ART
OF MEDICINE. 8vo. cloth, 8s.

DR. WEST.

LECTURES ON THE DISEASES OF WOMEN. 8vo. cloth, 10s. 6d.

MR. T. SPENCER WELLS, F.R.C.S.

PRACTICAL OBSERVATIONS ON GOUT AND ITS COMPLI-
CATIONS, and on the Treatment of Joints Stiffened by Gouty Deposits.　Foolscap 8vo. cloth, 5s.

MR. WHEELER.

HAND-BOOK OF ANATOMY FOR STUDENTS OF THE
FINE ARTS.　New Edition, with Engravings on Wood.　Fcap. 8vo., 2s. 6d.

DR. WHITEHEAD, F.R.C.S.

I.

ON THE TRANSMISSION FROM PARENT TO OFFSPRING
OF SOME FORMS OF DISEASE, AND OF MORBID TAINTS AND TENDENCIES.　Second Edition.　8vo. cloth, 10s. 6d.

II.

THE CAUSES AND TREATMENT OF ABORTION AND
STERILITY: being the result of an extended Practical Inquiry into the Physiological and Morbid Conditions of the Uterus, with reference especially to Leucorrhœal Affections, and the Diseases of Menstruation.　8vo. cloth, 12s.

DR. WILLIAMS, F.R.S.

PRINCIPLES OF MEDICINE: An Elementary View of the Causes,
Nature, Treatment, Diagnosis, and Prognosis, of Disease.　With brief Remarks on Hygienics, or the Preservation of Health.　The Third Edition.　8vo. cloth, 15s.

DR. JOSEPH WILLIAMS.

INSANITY: its Causes, Prevention, and Cure; including Apoplexy,
Epilepsy, and Congestion of the Brain.　Second Edition.　Post 8vo. cloth, 10s. 6d.

DR. J. HUME WILLIAMS.

UNSOUNDNESS OF MIND, IN ITS MEDICAL AND LEGAL
CONSIDERATIONS.　8vo. cloth, 7s. 6d.

DR. HENRY G. WRIGHT.

HEADACHES; their Causes and their Cure.　Second Edition.　Fcap. 8vo.
2s. 6d.

MR. ERASMUS WILSON, F.R.S.

I.

THE ANATOMIST'S VADE-MECUM: A SYSTEM OF HUMAN

ANATOMY. With numerous Illustrations on Wood. Seventh Edition. Foolscap 8vo. cloth, 12s. 6d.

II.

DISEASES OF THE SKIN: A Practical and Theoretical Treatise on

the DIAGNOSIS, PATHOLOGY, and TREATMENT OF CUTANEOUS DIS-EASES. Fourth Edition. 8vo. cloth, 16s.

THE SAME WORK; illustrated with finely executed Engravings on Steel, accurately coloured. 8vo. cloth, 34s.

III.

HEALTHY SKIN: A Treatise on the Management of the Skin and Hair

in relation to Health. Fifth Edition. Foolscap 8vo. 2s. 6d.

IV.

PORTRAITS OF DISEASES OF THE SKIN. Folio. Fasciculi I.

to XII., completing the Work. 20s. each.

V.

ON SYPHILIS, CONSTITUTIONAL AND HEREDITARY;

AND ON SYPHILITIC ERUPTIONS. With Four Coloured Plates. 8vo. cloth, 16s.

VI.

A THREE WEEKS' SCAMPER THROUGH THE SPAS OF

GERMANY AND BELGIUM, with an Appendix on the Nature and Uses of Mineral Waters. Post 8vo. cloth, 6s.

DR. FORBES WINSLOW, D.C.L. OXON.

I.

LETTSOMIAN LECTURES ON INSANITY. 8vo. cloth, 5s.

II.

A SYNOPSIS OF THE LAW OF LUNACY; as far as it relates

to the Organization and Management of Private Asylums for the Care and Treatment of the Insane. In the form of a Chart, varnished, mounted on canvas and rollers, price 6s.

DR. G. C. WITTSTEIN.

PRACTICAL PHARMACEUTICAL CHEMISTRY: An Explanation

of Chemical and Pharmaceutical Processes, with the Methods of Testing the Purity of the Preparations, deduced from Original Experiments. Translated from the Second German Edition, by STEPHEN DARBY. 18mo. cloth, 6s.

MR. YEARSLEY.

DEAFNESS PRACTICALLY ILLUSTRATED; being an Exposition

of Original Views as to the Causes and Treatment of Diseases of the Ear. Fifth Edition. Foolscap 8vo., 2s. 6d.

II.

ON THE ENLARGED TONSIL AND ELONGATED UVULA,

and other Morbid Conditions of the Throat. Sixth Edition. 8vo. cloth, 5s.

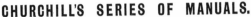

CHURCHILL'S SERIES OF MANUALS.

"We here give Mr. Churchill public thanks for the positive benefit conferred on the Medical Profession, by the series of beautiful and cheap Manuals which bear his imprint."— *British and Foreign Medical Review.*

AGGREGATE SALE 91,000 COPIES.

DR. BARLOW.
A MANUAL OF THE PRACTICE OF MEDICINE.
Foolscap 8vo. cloth, 12s. 6d.

DR. GOLDING BIRD, F.R.S., and CHARLES BROOKE, M.B. Cantab, F.R.S.
ELEMENTS OF NATURAL PHILOSOPHY;
Being an Experimental Introduction to the Study of the Physical Sciences. With numerous Illustrations on Wood. Fourth Edition. Fcap. 8vo. cloth, 12s. 6d.

DR. CARPENTER, F.R.S.
A MANUAL OF PHYSIOLOGY.
With numerous Illustrations on Steel and Wood. Third Edition. Fcap. 8vo. cloth, 12s. 6d.
BY THE SAME AUTHOR.
THE MICROSCOPE AND ITS REVELATIONS.
With numerous Engravings on Wood. Second Edition. Fcap. 8vo. cloth, 12s. 6d.

MR. FERGUSSON, F.R.S.E.
A SYSTEM OF PRACTICAL SURGERY.
With numerous Illustrations on Wood. Fourth Edition. Fcap. 8vo. cloth, 12s. 6d.

MR. FOWNES, PH.D., F.R.S.
A MANUAL OF CHEMISTRY.
With numerous Illustrations on Wood. Sixth Edition. Fcap. 8vo. cloth, 12s. 6d.

MR. WHARTON JONES, F.R.S.
A MANUAL OF OPHTHALMIC MEDICINE & SURGERY.
With Coloured Engravings on Steel, and Illustrations on Wood. Second Edition. Fcap. 8vo. cloth, 12s. 6d.

Dr. HANDFIELD JONES, F.R.S., & Dr. EDWARD H. SIEVEKING.
A MANUAL OF PATHOLOGICAL ANATOMY.
Illustrated with numerous Engravings on Wood. Foolscap 8vo., cloth, 12s. 6d.

DR. ROYLE, F.R.S., and DR. HEADLAND, F.L.S.
A MANUAL OF MATERIA-MEDICA.
With numerous Illustrations on Wood. Third Edition. Fcap. 8vo. cloth, 12s. 6d.

DR. ALFRED TAYLOR, F.R.S.
A MANUAL OF MEDICAL JURISPRUDENCE.
Fifth Edition. Fcap. 8vo. cloth, 12s. 6d,
BY THE SAME AUTHOR.
ON POISONS.
Fcap. 8vo. cloth, 12s. 6d.

MR. ERASMUS WILSON, F.R.S.
THE ANATOMIST'S VADE-MECUM;
A SYSTEM OF HUMAN ANATOMY. With numerous Illustrations on Wood. Seventh Edition. Fcap. 8vo. cloth, 12s. 6d.

Printed by W. BLANCHARD & SONS, 62, Millbank Street, Westminster.

This special edition of

ON MALFORMATIONS, &c.,
OF THE HUMAN HEART

By THOMAS B. PEACOCK, M.D.

*has been privately printed for members of
The Classics of Medicine Library by Halliday
Lithograph Company. Film was prepared
from an original 1858 edition, furnished to
the Publisher courtesy of the Francis A. Count-
way Library of Medicine. New type matter was
composed by Boro Typographers Inc. in De-
Vinne. The text paper was especially made for
this edition by the S.D. Warren Company. The
volume has been bound in genuine top grain
cowhide with endleaves in a marbled design
by the Tapley-Rutter Company, Bookbinders.
Edges are gilded and covers are brass-die
stamped in 22-karat gold. Cover stampings
and design of the edition by Daniel B. Bianchi
and Selma Ordewer.*

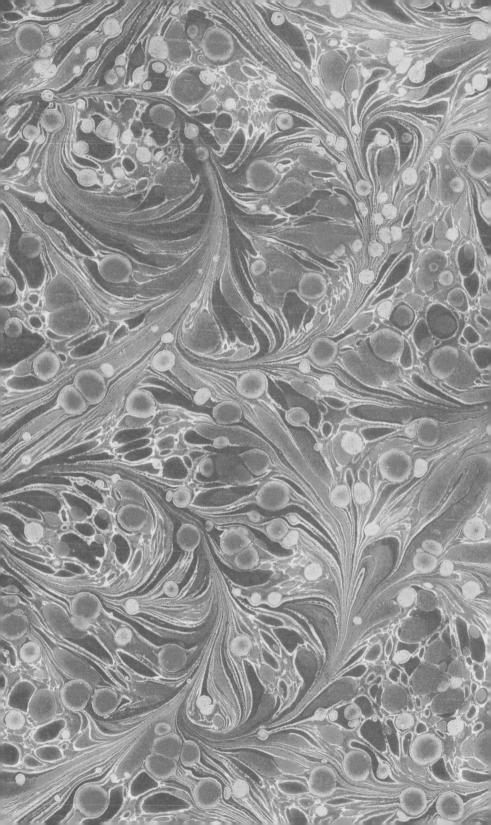